AIDS and the National Body

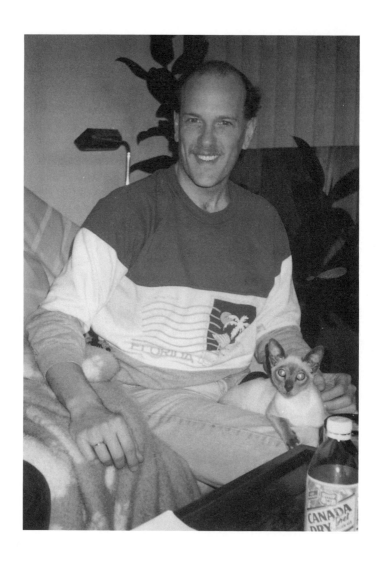

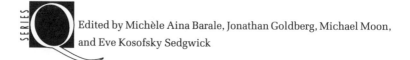

SERIES Q Edited by Michèle Aina Barale, Jonathan Goldberg, Michael Moon, and Eve Kosofsky Sedgwick

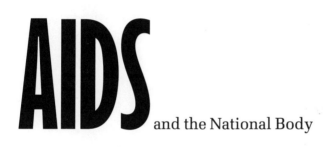and the National Body

Thomas E. Yingling

Edited, and with an introduction by Robyn Wiegman

Duke University Press   Durham & London 1997

© 1997 The Estate of Thomas E. Yingling

"Editor's Introduction," "The Burdens of One's Deeper Debts,"

"The Mortal Limits of Poetry and Criticism: Reading Yingling,

Reading Gunn," and "Caesura" © 1997 Duke University Press

All rights reserved

Printed in the United States of America on acid-free paper ∞

Typeset in Melior by Keystone Typesetting, Inc.

Acknowledgment of copyrights and Library of Congress

Cataloging-in-Publication Data appear on the last printed

page of this book.

The Dream Visitor

Approximately one month before the appearance of my first Kaposi's
sarcoma lesions, I had a dream in which I was visited by a figure.
He did not enjoin me to repent, as does the dream visitor in *Parting
Glances.* In fact, he had been dispatched with knowledge. There was
some important communication between him and me, but the issue
here was that he couldn't speak. This man was a Holocaust figure—he
was on his way to the trains: millions dead, and they all knew it, and
no one did anything. What I recall—in addition to the shabby dignity of
his demeanor—was the utter boundlessness of the injustice of whatever ignorance it was we were condemned to and by in our communication. AIDS had shifted from a question of morality to one of epistemology. Then, I am reading Wittgenstein, and I come across this: "Look
upon this tumor as a perfectly normal part of your body"—what is a
perfectly normal part of my body? AIDS had shifted to humor. But this
is the move one must make, and in order to do it, one must not "look
on" but *read,* and it is the question of reading with uncertain terms that
AIDS forces upon us. The whole business of the national body begins
here.

Contents

Knowledge Effects

The Stuttering I

Introduction

Robyn Wiegman

I shall never get you put together entirely.
—Sylvia Plath, "The Colossus"

When Tom Yingling died in 1992, he left no instructions, only an improperly signed will, a few pieces of furniture, a car, and a diversity of writing—poetry, lectures, essays, abstracts for books and papers, journal entries, letters to friends. He left the way people leave their houses to go to work in the morning. Of course he knew that he was dying, but as with each of us, he had a particular approach, a form and manner, to his personal grief. According to his own narrative, he had always struggled with postponement: not "coming out" until his early thirties, launching his academic career later in that decade, telling people who really mattered to him about his illness only at the end. He fretted over his relationship to time, to the significance, symbolically, emotionally, of how and when and if he would arrive. In this way, it seems to me, his death at the age of forty-two snuck up on him. He was not accustomed to being early.

I met Tom at the end of 1987. He was an Emerson Fellow in the English Department at Syracuse University, finishing a manuscript that the University of Chicago Press would publish as *Hart Crane and the Homosexual Text* (1990). He had been particularly active in the theory debates that accompanied the department's reformulation of its undergraduate curriculum, a process that abolished historical periodicity as the governing rubric and put in its place the organizing categories of "History, Theory, Politics." Tom found himself most often teaching courses under "politics," and one might characterize his critical practice at the time as a heady mixture of poststructuralist theory and postmodern Marxist ideology critique. He took from poststructuralism an attention to the discursive articulation of social relations, what he calls in *Hart Crane* "the placement of subjects in discourse" (2), and from Marxism what he cites as a concern for "the materiality of literary production and reception" (14).

After the completion of *Hart Crane* and with the decidedly material influence of his own HIV-positivity, diagnosed in 1989, Tom became increasingly suspicious of his earlier critical tendencies. The poststructuralist critique of the individual and of humanist notions of identity, essence, and experience—in short, the theoretical legacy of "social constructionism"—would not be wholly adequate to the way he wanted to think about the complexities of embodied identity, nor would a return to humanism suffice. While he found in psychoanalysis an interesting attempt to discuss the subjective contours of identity, Tom was finally too uncomfortable with the way theoretical practices were most often mastering methodologies for the critic's own claim to epistemological sovereignty. As the essays in this volume will demonstrate, Tom was increasingly drawn to a self-conscious critical practice that could handle the inability of the critic to finally and assuredly know.

One cannot help but to read such a critical turn away from ideology critique and certain assumptions of poststructuralism as a consequence of AIDS—both "my AIDS," as he describes it, and AIDS as a social relation. For Yingling, AIDS was the "disease that announces the end of identity" (15; this volume), and he meant this as much on the individual level as the national. In Tom's thinking, AIDS made palpable—to the point of psychic crisis—the irreconcilability of the body's materiality and our imaginary relation to it. He spoke compellingly of his own difficulty adjusting to the way HIV manifested itself in highly visible and swift changes, from the spread of Kaposi's sarcoma (KS) (first his leg, then chest, face, and arms) to weight and hair loss, bruising, bloating, and blindness. (Friends, doctors, even Tom, were shocked at the way the KS spread from its initial spot on his leg in February 1991 to nearly 90 percent of his body by July 1992. During the last week of life, he was blind from this aspect of his illness.) In literalizing the contradiction between the material and the imaginary body, AIDS interrupted the fantasy of "sameness" that underlies psychic holds on identity and the coherent "self." AIDS thus became for Yingling the literal and symbolic figure of the "non-identical"—that which could never be thought of as "itself" *and* that which undid the very fiction of the self.

Otherness as a condition of the constitution of the "self"—the misrecognition necessary to its own formation—is certainly not Yingling's invention. But the exploration of the way AIDS circumvents identity's fundamental repression is a crucial contribution to the critical discourse about the disease. More important still is Yingling's focus on "the national body"—the phrase he used to link the individual experience of AIDS to historical configurations of power, sexuality, capital, and identity. For Yingling, "the national body" references the social imaginary of identifications, desires, values, and practices that govern the legibility of the body in U.S. culture. "[N]ational identity," he writes in "Wittgenstein's Tumor," "requires an ideal conception of the body and a rejection of accommodation to Otherness" (25; this volume), and it does so in a context that understands "the ideal" as without disease in all senses: physical, moral, sexual—in short, as a normative and regulatory ideal. Exploring how that ideal functions, especially in popular discourses about HIV infection and AIDS, was for Yingling crucial to any critical engagement with the disease, drawing him into a conversation about the precise ways in which AIDS has been figured as anti-American: in its violation of heterosexually sanctioned erogenous zones, familial bonds, and social formations of privacy and pleasure, along with its narrative tropes of invasion, foreign bodies, and altered alterities.

I found "Wittgenstein's Tumor: AIDS and the National Body" under a stack of papers on the floor of Tom's home office after he died, covered with notes in handwritten scrawl; I have never found the disk version, though in looking for it I came across many other documents that have become of use to me here. "The Dream Visitor," which opens this volume, for instance, existed in a file by itself, titled by Yingling, on the same floppy with "Hope," a meditation on the meaning of his own professional life in the context of being HIV+. I have included such writing in this volume—along with poems, letters, and abstracts—in order to represent the tensions I read in Tom's work on the national body: the way AIDS figures as a critical—in all senses of the word—social condition and its individual interiorization. That Tom would be embarrassed by the exposure of the personal I do not doubt. The disease did embarrass him, not just in the national discourse of sexual shame that surrounds HIV transmission, but in the debilitating corporeal transformations it visited upon him. But it seems to me that Tom's focus on the national body—the last essay he would write—necessitates just such an exposure: when the legibility of one's own body is shorn from all imaginary relations, not only those governing national and personal identity, but those of desire, consumption, and labor as well.

These last issues—of consumption and labor—are perhaps less developed than the others in the keynote essay of this volume, but their significance for the meaning of living and writing with AIDS is profound. In discussing how the "national feeling for the body" is linked to commodity culture, Tom rather quickly notes in "Wittgenstein's Tumor" that "AIDS places one outside the circuits of that culture" (29; this volume). While he does not develop this idea much further, it is easy to see how the familiar image of the "wasted" AIDS body—the very cultural insistence on such an image as *the* predominant sign for the disease—emphasizes the point, as the body might be said to "fail" in both ways: it is no longer capable of labor (so-called meaningful or otherwise) or of entering the circuits of exchange necessary to the "pleasures" of commodity consumption. Expenditure—for drug treatments, high-cost medical practices and insurance policies, therapy—promises postponement, not pleasure. Likewise eating, so often a practice of pleasure, becomes for the person living with AIDS, or PLWA (and especially for Tom, who found immense satisfaction in food), a consumptive practice more indicative of the body's social and psychic abjection.

And what of labor? Tom doesn't say much directly about this in "Wittgenstein's Tumor" and yet the composite of essays offered here cannot escape their own bearing on the complexities of "work" for the PLWA. In the alienation that the severance from the national body engendered, in the contemplative posture of a man watching his body's material reformations, in his own personal engagement with identity's inscription within Western regimes of a mind/body split, Tom seemed to struggle—both for and against—the cultural function of work as a normalizing agency. During the last year of his life, he was director of graduate studies in English at Syracuse and a member of various dissertation and thesis committees. "Working with the grad students is extremely fulfilling—even in the face of the uncertainty of the future," he writes to an old friend, in a letter I've reprinted here. The work of the critic, on the other hand, "has not been of much importance to me at all: I finally get invitations to speak places (I'm supposed to go back to Penn to speak in January—something I always fantasized about) and I don't care anymore about academic writing and research" (11; this volume). And yet Tom would return seven months before he died to Penn, where he had attended graduate school in the mid-eighties, to deliver "Wittgenstein's Tumor," an essay he would continue to revise— from what I can tell—until at least early May 1992. He would also deliver versions of the essay at Cornell and Columbia; produce an abstract for a Modern Language Association panel that last spring (see "AIDS, Confession, and Theory" in this volume); continue to draft "Fetishism, Identity, Politics," begun a year earlier (also included here); and tinker with his essays on lyric poetry and the politics of the canon (see "The Stuttering I" and "Theory and Debate over Canon" in this volume).

Yingling's lack of "care" did not translate, then, into a cessation of academic production; rather his relation to that production and the meaning of that production ceased to signify apart from "my AIDS." The materiality of the illness infected, if you will, not simply his relationship to time, but the hierarchies of meaning with which life was itself invested. The protocols of academic work that privilege the individual as an intellectual mind, the lengthy cycle of writing/revision/ submission/publication, the circulation of oneself at conferences and symposia, the various routines associated with the crafting of a "national" reputation: these were no longer the conceptual contours of his identifications, the manner through which he placed himself in time. Instead, he seems to have sought—what? not solace nor comfort, certainly not fulfillment, perhaps just some kind of maintenance—in his relationship to the everyday, a suspension of the academic's vested interest in his (or her) future arrival. "I don't regret the choices I made in getting into this," he writes, "it just no longer seems like the most important aspect of life" (11; this volume).

It is consistent with his own complex sentiments about academic production that Tom made few plans while still alive concerning the future handling of his scholarship. While he named me as his literary executive in a will prepared in 1991, he never managed to legally sign it. We had no conversations in which he provided organizing directions or conceptual frameworks for the essays, published and unpublished, that were never collected; he located no disks, gathered together no errant manuscripts. I have—it must be said—insinuated myself into the task of assembling his writing, partly as mourning, partly as emblem of intellectual respect, and partly to satisfy my own need to participate in a politics of surviving.

Others have joined me in this—Michael Awkward, David Román, Robert L. Caserio, and Stephen Melville—each of whom knew Tom in differing ways and who bring compellingly different conversations to interact with his work in this anthology. Awkward uses both personal narrative and literary critical strategies to engage Tom's analysis of Robert Mapplethorpe's photographs of black men, challenging the way identity-based theory has overinvested in social categories (of gender, race, sexuality) to define political epistemologies and psychic interiorities. Román writes in response to Yingling's assertion that gay studies has achieved academic legitimacy by locating the elisions and limitations of the contemporary formation of sexuality studies. Caserio provides a critical engagement with Yingling's *Hart Crane and the Homosexual Text,* carrying into the present an argument about poetry and theory that he had only just begun with Tom before he died. And Melville closes this volume with a consideration of what AIDS has (and does not have) to teach us—about community, loss, and our own "out, living" (172; this volume). In reflecting on Tom's own writing and on the contexts that give rise to this collection, the essays by contemporary scholars extend the polyvocality we find in Tom's work, being at once personal narrative, literary criticism, social commentary, and critical theory. They embody, if you will, the breadth of Tom's own critical dialogues—moving from visual culture to the canonical formation of gay and lesbian studies, to twentieth-century American poetry, to the politics of the academy—and they do so by taking up quite explicitly the way AIDS, "that word by itself" (58; this volume), is the critical center of this book.

Approximately two weeks after Tom died, I had a dream in which he visited me. The scene was the hospital room. I was sitting in a green chair. Tom's KS had begun to disappear; he was no longer blind. When he told me he had to leave, the hospital door swung open and, as I watched him exit, he turned into a young boy with a perfectly normal body. The dream was more comforting to me then than it is now, with its compensatory fantasy that AIDS had lost its power over him. I've read enough Yingling to become distrustful of the resurrection of the imaginary body, and I do not want to find in his death a way to manage my own relationship to AIDS as psychic closure. Indeed, it seems to me that the critical importance of this volume lies precisely in its ability to render the contradictory power of AIDS.

September 1, 1991

Dear ——

Your letter arrived about two or three weeks ago, and I've put off answering because I haven't wanted to deal with the issues you raised. To
make a very long and very complicated story short, I became symptomatic of AIDS in February of this year. I have Kaposi's sarcoma, which is
the skin cancer associated with HIV. I've spent the summer trying to
work some chemotherapy (an injection of interferon that I do once a
day), but the success has been negligible and the side effects fairly
debilitating (I spent June and July on the couch watching cable, trying
to keep the room from spinning). But the lesions continue to spread. It
doesn't appear that KS is metastatic: it simply pops up spontaneously
anywhere on the body: the only seriously threatening sites are all internal, and we're trying to slow its spread and (hopefully) keep it all
external. But no one knows with this disease; it seems that it just goes
wherever it wants, and while the drugs may interfere with the progres-
sion toward serious illness, they don't seem able really to reverse or
halt it.

Needless to say, coping with all of this has been weird and awful. As
you probably know from your mother's illness, the psychological pro-

cess is more intense than the physical. I've known for two years (yesterday) that I was HIV+; I've been on AZT for almost two years. The lesions (my only prominent symptom of AIDS so far) appeared in February and were confirmed through biopsy in March. By April, I was a basket case. Then I got really run down in May—and once school was over, we (the doctor and I) decided to try the interferon treatment since the KS appeared to be advancing fairly aggressively.

I suppose I might have told you all of this years ago, but I didn't tell anyone except two or three people. It is still information I can't (psychically can't) share with everyone; I'm still working (the department is putting me up for promotion this year), and I want my life to retain whatever normal patterns it can for as long as possible, and it just seems to me that people's knowing would change things too much. It's not that I'm afraid of being run out of town or anything, but it doesn't seem to be the business of people who know nothing about the illness and care little or nothing about me. I want to avoid what I know has already happened: people who don't talk to me who talk about me.

This is the strangest letter I've ever written to anyone. I don't think any of it follows coherently; it may just be venting, and while that's great it also means I'm skipping over important stuff as I go along. Let me say first of all that not every day is hell or doom for me: I'm living with my friend Randy (also positive but still quite strong and healthy) and another friend in a huge and gorgeous house in Syracuse. They are so helpful and supportive, and our domestic contentment is one of the most important things to me right now. There are days, of course, when I want to run away even from them, but basically I'm trying to work with the disease and not let it control me. I've been in a support group for two years, which is often a life-raft. But it is hard: and the hardest part is that I don't know if I'll make it for one more year or for a decade or more. I truly believe that some people will survive this epidemic; but I also know that most of us won't, and I try to be both realistic and hopeful (a tough seesaw act).

Anyway, I get very sentimental these days—seeing all the wonderful people I've had in my life and wondering if I've done the right thing by them. Missing them. Grieving, I guess. And of course wondering "why me?" and trying to fix (retroactively) what isn't really broken (me, friendships, the past). We watched *Beaches* last night and the scene that stays with me most is when Barbara Hershey can't find a picture of her mother's hands: how insistently she needs this object (the picture)—with an irrational passion—as if that were going to give her the answer to all the unanswerable questions.

More than anything else, I feel those unanswerable questions these days, and a strong pull toward a certain reverence for life that I haven't felt for years: to allow myself to feel reverence (not fake religion or panicked bargaining with god, but a mysterious recognition that might almost promise contentment). That means as well, of course, that work has not been of much importance to me at all: I finally get invitations to speak places (I'm supposed to go back to Penn to speak in January—something I always fantasized about) and I don't care anymore about academic writing and research. But that has something to do with this un-answerability: as academics we're forced to act as if we have all the answers. The rewarding of aggressive hostility in the profession has come to bother me immensely: none of it is worth the ill-feeling, the intrigues, the inflated sense of purpose. I don't regret the choices I made in getting into this, it just no longer seems like the most important aspect of life (middle-age crisis strikes Central New York PWA—film at eleven).

Through all of this I have maintained (and continue to try to maintain) a sense of humor—perhaps a little more sardonic at times. I refuse to live thinking only about "the end." So I'm director of graduate studies this year in the department (only teaching one course per semester). Working with the grad students is extremely fulfilling—even in the face of the uncertainty of the future.

I'm beginning to see that at this point, I'm writing more for myself than for you, so perhaps I should stop . . . I want you to know that I am basically optimistic—if not about living to 100, at least about what my life *still* is and can be. So although this letter may shock and sadden, please be sure that I'm hanging in there. Call or write soon,

Tom

Reading with Uncertain Terms

The Oncology of Ontology

On first reading a certain work by Derrida, I mistook the word "ontology" for "oncology." That is the *thing* of AIDS, it is the signifier through which we understand the cancer of being, the oncology of ontology—not only in its threat to our being, its announcement that we are moving toward non-being, indeed are already inscribed with it, in it. But also that it is itself deeply not-identical, never quite the same, appearing under different guises, none of which is a disguise, following circuitous routes into visibility and action. It is the disease that announces the end of identity.

   ... Since its naming, AIDS has been presented to us as both physically and figurally overwhelming, as virtually irresistible in its meanings. And most of that figuration has centered on linking AIDS either directly or metaphorically to desire—either through homosexuality or drug use, both of which stand in synecdochically for a longer list of policed activities. That those two activities in particular could come to signify AIDS is itself a sleight of hand we might investigate, and most of our thinking about AIDS in psychoanalytic terms has turned on how desire is immobilized (and therefore mobilized) in discourses about it: we can read the political unconscious of Jesse Helms (his literal unconscious being too excrescent to repay any attention); we can read American anxieties about nonmonogamous, heterosexual sexual activity; we can analyze the Other of American televisual domains (the African American, the Latin, the homeless, the sick in general: how can you be a consumer when you are yourself consumed with illness?).

But more than the politics of desire is at stake in thinking about AIDS: in fact, it may well be that AIDS has said more about identity in our culture than it could ever say about desire. More specifically, we might ask—through Lacan and others—about the mirror stage and the relation of the "I" to its body, for we encounter in living with AIDS the production of non-subjects, people for whom the mirroring illusions of discourse are broken: the host body in this case continually reminds its subject—with every glance in the mirror—of the distance between the "I" and its lesions, and of the fact that the lesions may not be subsumed into any transcendence; thus, one of the important discursive moves from the beginning has been the insistence on the designation "person with AIDS." The struggle in living with AIDS is to produce a discourse adequate to an experience that is not deterritorialization (the term Gilles Deleuze and Félix Guattari use to describe the flow of desiring-production beyond the categories inscribed in the subject) but reterritorialization (their term for the new "form" or convention desire produces; its making): a new identity, a new codification and damming of the flow of desire is offered in the body of the person with AIDS, but that subject has in fact been emptied of desire.

It is thus that Kafka's work—in which our reading shuttles among fields we might call the body of desiring-production, its denial, and the legislation of identity—becomes allegorical to living with AIDS and finally more telling in its allegory than referential texts like *Longtime Companion* or *Parting Glances*. Texts of body loss (see here as well *The Fly* and *The Elephant Man*) are allegorical for AIDS not only because they place in motion alienation from a body that no longer seems to house a subject, but also because they foreground the impossibility of speaking the condition of loss being written into (and onto) the body. So it is not desire that is in question, but identity: the whole problem of a disappearing body, of a body quite literally shitting itself away. That is AIDS.

Wittgenstein's Tumor:
AIDS and the National Body

Toward the end of "Modernity—An incomplete project," the essay he delivered on the occasion of receiving the Adorno Prize from the city of Frankfurt in 1980, Jürgen Habermas reminds us of the differing function and meaning the same object may solicit in different social contexts. He suggests that while an aesthetic object may call forth one reading from the expert or critic, there is too little homogeneity in modern culture to guarantee that its entry into the life experience of that culture will be congruent with the critic's reading:

> as soon as such an experience [an aesthetic experience] is used to illuminate a life-historical situation and is related to life problems, it enters into a language game which is no longer that of the aesthetic critic. The aesthetic experience then not only renews the interpretation of our needs in whose light we perceive the world. It permeates as well our cognitive significations and our normative expectations and changes the manner in which all these moments refer to one another. (13)

Citing the dual demand within bourgeois culture that one be both a critical respondent to art and a consumer subject to the pleasure of fashion, Habermas rejects the aesthetic experience as a means toward meaningful social change, as a site for the completion of modernity's project of pursuing a rational human culture. We might borrow this Habermasian notion as a way to work into the question of what has gone wrong in American culture's lukewarm response to AIDS, where the "experts" (and critics) have found themselves unable to effect meaningful social change despite their expertise, their warnings, and their seemingly endless labor. In fact, Habermas's essay presents a number of interesting prospects in this regard: his use of Weber is a perfect place to begin to think about how the AIDS epidemic has been inscribed in dominant culture in a way that preserves the seeming autonomy of such fields as the scientific, the moral, and the aesthetic (that autonomy being, according to Weber, one of the legacies of modern industrial capitalism), so that one is invited to assume (as George Bush and other government leaders seem to) that research continues at its own pace (how can you hurry truth?), that the lay public cares deeply and can surfeit its fear and assuage its failure through aesthetic texts like *Longtime Companion* (1990), and that the moral issues of AIDS still turn on questions of condom distribution in schools and less on care and treatment of PWAs—or, more significantly, that moral issues are destined to remain indeterminate in a diverse culture such as America. One need not be a believer in Habermas's dream of a perfectly reintegrated, postcapitalist culture in order to begin to trace how a successful campaign of response to AIDS needs to move across the false autonomy of these realms.

But this may also be the expert's position, largely lost on the culture as it expresses AIDS in its dominant modes; in other words, while writers like Simon Watney or Cindy Patton might be able convincingly to demonstrate a detrimental link between the false neutrality of science and the political realities of living with AIDS, that will probably have very little impact on those school board members who are reaching a decision about AIDS education in some small town in upstate New York. This is one of the reasons for some skepticism in the HIV community about the way in which the media have taken up figures like Magic Johnson and Kimberley Bergalis: relatively sophisticated readings of AIDS as signifier or as social fact have received none of the attention recently lavished on these two despite their seeming lack of knowledge about the epidemic.[1] Unfortunately, one must say that their entry into AIDS discourses has always bordered on the specular (this perhaps against their own best intentions), making AIDS "real" by circulating images that refer not to the complex interdiscursive challenges of the disease but to other, familiar images: in the Johnson case these images are of sport, in Bergalis it is the popular image of the weak, debilitated AIDS victim, of the suffering terminal patient. If writers like Baudrillard are correct, and the media operate at the level of a hyper-reality, circulating images and information without reference to the production of meaning, then sports entertainment is one of the supreme modes of that circulation in our culture: the question of meaning is never even staged (as it may be, for instance, in other areas of the news); we are simply invited to bask in the play of images that refer only to images in a system underwritten by their seductive appeal. We might note as well that sport functions interestingly to secure a sense of national identity: in the nineteenth century, production and commerce defined the relation between regions in America. Now, in an era of multinational corporate structures, it is more likely that Buffalo is linked to Washington, D.C. only through the Super Bowl (we see the older model parodied in odd little practices like the wager of a bushel of lobsters and a bushel of oranges between governors of states whose "teams" will compete on the athletic field). What happens when AIDS invades that system? It is literally unthinkable in the terms usually at play there; thus, Magic has to be removed from the system.

The media have used both Bergalis and Johnson largely to evoke emotional response. Thus, while Bergalis's case appeared to open debate about the ethics or morality of certain medical practices—and therefore to offer a potential bridge to the false autonomy of science and ethics as they have been constructed around this disease—we really need rather to read her position in a nationally circulated and nationally inspired narrative of fear and pity that leveled any impact her illness and death might have had on public health debates and made of her crusade mostly an enactment of pathos. Expert only in suffering innocence (truly the AIDS victim), Bergalis signified for America one of the tragic dimensions of the epidemic, but the spectacle she provided would remain trapped in the realm of the aesthetic. The Magic Johnson case is slightly different. By working with the experts rather than against them, as Bergalis did, Johnson allows himself to be presented as someone with the potential to have a significant impact on the legitimation of AIDS and HIV as a speakable concern, especially among the African American, teen, and heterosexual populations.

And there is heartening evidence that he may remain the occasion for some rational debate about safe sex and/or abstinence as appropriate preventives of transmission (although after his appointment to the president's AIDS commission, he evidently added the advice of abstinence to his routine statements about HIV). But while the figure at its center is heroic rather than pathetic, here too we are confronted mostly with an aesthetic text designed to elicit feeling from an audience: one of our champions will perhaps be cut down in his prime; it is Lou Gehrig, Ajax, or Achilles.

Perhaps the most telling effect in both these instances is the role irony plays in their construction. In both instances we are treated to a spectacle of the unexpected. The Bergalis story is drenched in irony: not only is she a young woman, and women, of course, are not at risk from AIDS, but more importantly, her case became so newsworthy because a simple medical procedure (routine dental care) evidently was the origin of her infection. Her appearance before a Congressional committee was likewise represented as ironic in the sense that her own death was imminent and yet she sought to protect others from such incidental infection—perhaps measures could be taken to save lives in the future, but those measures would be too late to save Kimberley Bergalis. And the final irony, the issue that threatened to bring down the entire edifice of HIV rights, was the "failure" of the CDC—that watchdog agency of public health—to support her position. The Johnson case also reads as deeply ironic: athletic heroes simply are not at risk from AIDS, and the discourse around their accomplishments is completely incompatible with representations of AIDS. Johnson has also been adamant in his refusal to admit any homosexuality as a possible source for his infection, making him a truly exceptional figure for HIV infection. Another drug-user, another homosexual, another sex-worker: their contraction of HIV is not newsworthy—there is simply nothing to tell the public about people with AIDS until it appears in some venue thought immune to it (as *People* magazine put it in covering the Johnson story, "Most of us are not homosexuals; most of us are not intravenous drug users" [Alexander and Benet 59]—as if most of us *were* professional athletes!). Most significantly, Johnson had always signified for American culture a Huck Finn–like likeability: his boyish grin, the seemingly bottomless reservoir of a good-humored nature (and this alongside an obvious competitiveness). So "nice" was he that Johnson had, in fact, helped to resurrect professional basketball among white audiences in the seventies and eighties when polls had shown the dominance of African American players to have alienated large segments of white America. So the irony here is that Johnson, the perpetual adolescent in an adult body, the player who had no ill will toward his rivals yet usually prevailed over them, the Negro who could be trusted—Johnson was a "nice" person, and AIDS happened only to people who weren't "nice" and had courted disaster or failure in their personal lives.

What allows irony to work, of course, is a traditional notion that texts are stable and expectations clear *if* reversible; irony sets a limit to the instability of reading by staging closure as a choice between alternatives, each of which is complete. Irony thus provides an epistemological security rather than a radical textual opening. Rather than lead to questions about the grounds of reading, the seeming undecidability of irony becomes the key to a new stability. Thus, in the name of telling us something about AIDS, the media allows us to read AIDS—the most destabilizing social question of the last decade—through a set of stable discourses. Thus, in the Bergalis case—despite differing interpretations on the issue of whether medical personnel ought to tell clients of an HIV infection—it is assumed that there must be some right answer to the questions raised, that each side of the debate is reading the same text, and that such readings—and the text of AIDS itself as it is presented—spring not from an interested position but from a certifiable relation to truth. The multiplicity of those discourses does not, in fact, destabilize our reading practices or our relation to the disease; it simply says there are multiple perspectives, that each of them is clear, and that each presents some legitimate claim on our attention. The undecidability of irony on the emotional level becomes in this case an aesthetic strategy that mirrors the unresolvable nature of AIDS as a social ill.

But this shouldn't really surprise us. If it is not presented as a scientific issue or as a debate over some aspect of morality, AIDS is presented most often through the conventions of the human interest story, and most human interest stories—when they touch on "the controversial"—are constructed to ensure an emotional response as the only certain response to an irresolvable social problem that calls forth numerous other *un*certain responses. So what do I want? Would I rather there be no coverage of Magic Johnson? Certainly not. AIDS activism has lobbied for years for more public discourse about the disease, and now we seem to receive that; and government is spending—according to George Bush—more on AIDS research than on any other medical problem; so what do we want?

AIDS discourse for the first decade of the epidemic was consumed by the problem of meaning: what did AIDS mean as a social, historical event, and what did it mean to be a person with AIDS? Virtually all of the activity around the illness was bent on one goal (after, of course, the goal of education and prevention of infection): to secure a subjectivity for the person with AIDS that was not simply an erasure of his or her previous subjectivity, that did not simply read the illness as the end of meaning. Thus, we felt (I think) as though our task—and this we represented to ourselves in fairly heroic terms—was to wrest from dominant culture the wholly negative if not annihilative representation of HIV infection and AIDS, and to construct in its stead a discourse of empowerment, meaning, and possibility. And because of the historical conditions of the appearance of AIDS in the West, this was linked to a discursive explosion around the question of homosexuality: to effectively intervene in ignorant responses to AIDS, the institutional homophobia (particularly of America and Britain) had to be addressed and exposed (the best of this work remains Simon Watney's *Policing Desire*). That task has met with relative success, but we are still confronted on every side by a culture that has failed to integrate HIV and AIDS into its life experience (and I should say here that when I use a term like "experience" I mean that to signify a complex semiotic and dialectical process, not simply an unmediated knowledge of self or other). I want to suggest that we need a third phase response to AIDS: if phase one was pre-AZT and consisted mostly of emergency triage, phase two was post-AZT and consisted mostly of working *with* (or protesting against) researchers, pharmaceutical companies, and government agencies. Phase three needs to continue the pressure of phase two while expanding its frame of reference to address other cultural questions. We see how this has happened already with the birth of groups like Queer Nation, but I want to make this explicit: it is not enough to struggle to change the meaning of AIDS; we must begin to change that culture in which AIDS takes its meaning. This is where gay and lesbian academic work still can make a difference—because the culture in which AIDS takes its meaning (in America, at least) has read it as equivalent to homosexuality and has misread *that* with a criminal strength. More importantly, only gay and lesbian studies is positioned to continue the strong critique of that wholesale institutionalized homophobia that has largely determined the parameters of our thinking about sexuality.

In order to begin to make the call for such change less empty or obligatory, I want to turn to an unlikely text: Ludwig Wittgenstein's *Culture and Value,* and to a 1931 journal entry printed there. Wittgenstein, one of the gay modernists of Cambridge, is the subject of a recent critical biography that refused to take seriously the notion that sexual identity is a central component of subjectivity. As in the battle over Langston Hughes's sexuality—where one side (epitomized by the Rampersad biography and its squeamishness about Hughes's sexual history) seeks to deny the relevance if not the existence of homosexual desire in Hughes and the other side (let's say Isaac Julien or Essex Hemphill) presents Hughes as a symbol for the closeting of black male sexuality in white culture[2]—Wittgenstein's biographers have largely denied or minimized questions about desire in their reading of his work. The question of Wittgenstein's sexual identity is thought to sully his otherwise important contributions to philosophy, and his own deep repression of sexual questions in his writing—and his reported guilt over homosexual desire—both facilitate the argument that this has no impact on how we might most legitimately read his philosophy. We will return to this in a few moments, but for now, I would remind you that Wittgenstein died of cancer in 1951, making the following passage somewhat uncanny:

> "Look on this tumour as a perfectly normal part of your body!" Can one do that, to order? Do I have the power to decide at will to have, or not to have, an ideal conception of my body?
> ... We may say: people can only regard this tumour as a natural part of the body if their whole feeling for the body changes (if the whole national feeling for the body changes). Otherwise the best they can do is *put up with* it.
> You can expect an individual man to display this sort of tolerance, or else to disregard such things; but you cannot expect this of a nation, because it is precisely not disregarding such things that makes it a nation. I.e. there is a contradiction in expecting someone *both* to retain his former aesthetic feeling for the body and *also* to make the tumour welcome. (Wittgenstein 20e–21e)

There is a contradiction here: on the one hand, Wittgenstein tells us that one can't incorporate the tumor through strategies of accommodation; it will remain forever foreign to the self since the only language game one might invent for making the tumor a perfectly normal part of the body would be so private as to constitute what we would call an abnormal response. Wittgenstein is clear by this point in his life that language is a social act, that we may not simply use it to our own ends and that it is, in fact, often more determining of us than we of it; thus, one cannot look on the tumor—or any other object—in a willful manner if one hopes to reach some understanding of it:

> what makes a subject hard to understand—if it's something signifi-cant and important—is not that before you can understand it you need to be specially trained in abstruse matters, but the contrast between understanding the subject and what most people *want* to see. Because of this the very things which are most obvious may become the hardest of all to understand. What has to be overcome is a difficulty having to do with the will, rather than with the intellect. (17e)

On the other hand, Wittgenstein suggests that we might expect an individual to display a kind of tolerance toward the change in his body such that some truce with difference could be effected: but this is not a complete emotional or epistemological rapprochement—it is simply "the best they can do" to "*put up with* it," to allow it to stand in its difference. But there is perhaps a more crucial contradiction in Witt-genstein's equivocation about how the will might play in this matter, about whether or not "I"—or anyone—could have the power to decide to have—or not to have—an ideal conception of my body. The answer to this would seem a fairly strong "no," that larger culture forces deter-mine the ground of such attitudes. But *some* shift can occur in one's thinking if one begins to question cultural norms.

Somehow these questions turn for Wittgenstein on the prospect of national culture and identity, and in order to explain this, I should perhaps say that I have elided part of this passage, that disease here has a double valence. Following the first three sentences quoted above, we find a paragraph on a different kind of difference that may help explain Wittgenstein's curious assertion that the refusal of disease is essential to nationhood:

> Within the history of the peoples of Europe the history of the Jews is not treated as circumstantially as their intervention in European affairs would actually merit, because within this history they are experienced as a sort of disease, and anomaly, and no one wants to

put a disease on the same level as normal life [and no one wants to speak of a disease as if it had the same rights as healthy bodily processes (even painful ones)]. (20e)

We can just as easily imagine "queer" in place of "Jew" in this passage, but in writing of Jewish European history as disease, Wittgenstein seems to be responding to the rhetoric of National Socialism. Our reading of this passage should not stop at the simple solution of seeing disease as a cover signifier for "Jew," however: there is a national feeling for the body that is simply racist ideology but there is also a national feeling for the body that has to do with how our culture reads corporeality, physical competence, and health in general (each possibly inflected by racial discourse but not exhausted by it). Perhaps we need to take seriously Wittgenstein's suggestion that national identity requires an ideal conception of the body and a rejection of accommodation to Otherness.

The question we need to pursue turns on how the American feeling for the body inscribes disease as foreign and allows AIDS to be read therefore as anti-American. Before we turn to the question of the national feeling for the body, however, I would like to make a few remarks about the impact of AIDS on our thinking about the subject, for Wittgenstein's journal entry reminds us that the subject's self-relation is mediated, requiring us either to forgo rhetoric of a "Me" distinct from a "not-Me" or to open the term to a semiotic or dialectical reading. This would seem to be the impact of recent gay and lesbian theory as well, which has instructed us to question the very paradigm of identity that has allowed gays and lesbians to self-identify: Ed Cohen, among others, has written about the screen of sameness that underwrites the "we" of gay and lesbian political discourse, questioning how the categories of identity politics operate on an exclusionary principle similar to that which minority peoples have always had to work against and that imagines some essential condition of being signifiable as gay, lesbian, etcetera (see Cohen). Judith Roof has claimed that the paradigms of gay male subjectivity have been used to signify lesbian subjects, to turn them into sodomizing men, and Judith Butler, who has perhaps gone further than anyone else in reading identity as imitative and performative rather than constitutive, likewise considers any notion of the subject to be always already masculine (thus, her rejection of certain historical principles of feminism) (see Roof; Butler, *Gender Trouble*). Because of the way in which it parodies the very idea of origin and essence, drag becomes one of the privileged figures of identity for her, and in the rebirth of street theater around AIDS (in ACT UP, Queer Nation, PISD, and other group actions) we have seen the notion of politico-aesthetic performance resurrected with a vengeance.

But if we have sound intellectual and political reasons to be suspicious about the cultural and epistemological work performed in the name of the subject, we must also see that AIDS work has required construction of a juridical and social subject denominated "person with AIDS": in order to secure various entitlements (confidentiality as a principle of the ethics of the epidemic; funding for treatment and testing) and in order to resist the pressure to read AIDS only as the end of subjectivity and the loss of personal meaning, it has been absolutely necessary to make truck with the enemy and work with such categories as "intravenous drug-injector," "homosexual male," "person with AIDS," and "African American" as if the people meant to be covered by such phrases were actually named by them. But this is impossible. As Eve Sedgwick has pointed out in writing about the poverty of academic language in its description of such things as race, class, and sexual identity,[3] such terms hardly even begin to name the differences among us, so that one intravenous drug-injector may live homeless on the street, and one may live in the wealthiest section of the city. Choice of drugs, mode of access to those drugs, and specific practices in the use of those drugs may vary widely for different people all meant to be covered by this one term. And the category "person with AIDS" can be most empowering when least dominant: people living successfully with AIDS most often learn that they cannot escape the medical, juridical, and social category that marks them as diseased but that their resistance to the potentially negative effects of identification through AIDS is linked to how much they can refuse AIDS as a totalizing condition of being. To be able still to be a teacher, a student, an actor, a wife, lover, or child, a Republican or a Democrat, are all essential to a balanced response to diagnosis (this, too, is what made the figure of Kimberley Bergalis so pathetic: there was no frame of reference except her illness).

This is one of the crucial differences between commercial films like *An Early Frost* or *Longtime Companion,* both of which have been hailed for their ground-breaking representation of AIDS—one on television, the other in theaters—and an independent film like *Parting Glances.*[4] Both *An Early Frost* and *Longtime Companion* offer us the spectacle of how contraction of AIDS affects the bourgeois subject whose crisis is at the center of the narrative—in *An Early Frost* this is a young Chicago stockbroker whose family knows nothing of his homosexuality and who seems himself to know nothing about AIDS (he fails to read early signs like nightsweats and the incipient cough of pneumocystis as anything other than a flu); in *Longtime Companion* this involves a circle of friends in New York City who have lived, what we might call for want of a better term, the Fire Island life. The affluence of the central figures in both texts has been noted before, as has the fact that *An Early Frost*, cast as a family melodrama, seems to focus more on the family's (especially the father's) inability to name and accept the homosexuality of the son, rather than on the illness (we see Aiden Quinn, the son, in moments of illness, but the real burden of AIDS is enacted by a stereotypical "faggot," an unrepentant, bitter, impoverished, and lonely person with AIDS he meets in the hospital). *Longtime Companion* does, in this respect, have the virtue of representing AIDS as a communal rather than familial problem and of acknowledging the work gay people have done in caring for those with the disease. But in both instances we are invited to read AIDS mostly as the tumor that cannot be accommodated, as the end to what Michael Warner has called the "uniquely valuable subjectivity, the limitless self-formation and non-ascetic pleasures" that ground Americans' self-relations ("Walden's Erotic Economy" 173).

Parting Glances, on the other hand, offers us a completely different representation of AIDS and of the person with AIDS, making its AIDS character, Nick, seem at first almost incidental to a narrative in which "parting" will refer to Robert and John, lovers whose relationship is threatened by Robert's need to spend a year overseas on business. In the end, that parting does not occur, but Nick's illness brings us another sense of the potential partings that hover always between gay friends, and the film ends with another kind of parting glance, this a literal trashing and symbolic reading of the Fire Island life depicted in *Longtime Companion*—only the symbolic reading here constructs that world as fat and ridiculous. Unlike *An Early Frost* and *Longtime Companion,* both of which work to liberalize our attitude toward homosexuality by presenting bourgeois gay couples whose love for one another establishes their sameness to bourgeois heterosexual couples, *Parting Glances* does not work as a love story in the usual sense. While Robert and John have a relationship in which we as viewers are meant to invest, John explains to Nick in one of the film's most touching moments that it has always been him that he has loved, and other moments in the film reinforce our sense that desire circulates rather than settling in this text, that bodies move against one another (as at a party, as in dancing), and one cannot place a limit on their possible relations. Nick, whose character is defined by excess rather than absence (he is a rock singer, and the one piece we see of his is a video entitled "I'm only in it for the drugs"), refuses repentance as the appropriate response to his AIDS diagnosis. Unlike *An Early Frost*, this is not a narrative of Oedipal forgiveness, and when—in a parody of *Amadeus*—he is visited by a figure of doom linked intertextually to the father, saying only "Repent!" Nick throws a keyboard at him. Finally, Nick retains a sexual energy lost to melodramatic mourning in *An Early Frost* and *Longtime Companion;* rejecting suicide at the movie's close, Nick seems nevertheless to have incorporated knowledge of his death into life in a way that Bataille might approve, and to have moved the question of subjectivity around AIDS from one of hopeless loss to one of exuberant expenditure. Perhaps because the film celebrates a noninstrumental relation between the body and culture (all those marked by instrumentality are sexual and emotional pariahs), AIDS can become not the totalized moment of the subject's erasure, but another factor in a dance marked equally by death and desire.

This returns us to the question of what "the national feeling for the body" might be and how that might determine part of our thinking about AIDS. This is hardly an unexplored topic in American studies, of course: from Cooper on in the literature of the United States and at least since Fiedler, we have been aware of the peculiar parameters of the masculine subject offered in the name of "the American." Lauren Berlant has recently written of the paradox of privilege and disembodiment that defines the ideal of American citizenship: "if in practice the liberal political public sphere protects and privileges the [abstract] 'person's' racial and gendered embodiment [white, male], one effect of these privileges is to appear to be disembodied or abstract while retaining cultural authority. . . . In American culture . . . public embodiment is in itself a sign of inadequacy to proper citizenship" ("National Brands" 113–14). Thus, according to Berlant, women and people of color are always marked as inadequate and/or different because their identity is confirmed by the visibility of their bodily difference and by their social definition through the category of embodiment. Certainly we can include here people with AIDS, often physically marked by lesions, by wasting syndrome, by a T-shirt that reads "living with AIDS," and by a necessarily renewed knowledge of how fragile and

tenuous embodiment can be. This never-again-to-be disembodied subject thus typifies Wittgenstein's point about how an individual might
accommodate illness but a nation may not: it is in the self-definition of
the national to reject not only disease but the very notion of embodiment it recalls. Klaus Theweleit's *Male Fantasies* traces the burden of
such thinking in pre-Nazi ideology, suggesting that anything fluid,
feminine, or collective had to be disavowed by the masculine subject,
and if we are tempted to think that our culture's more recent interest in
the male body (in figures like Schwarzenegger or Stallone) recommends the masculine as a category of embodiment as well, we need
only see how the narratives they anchor celebrate the masculine subject's ability to transcend embodiment: wounds do not identify the
body as a surface inscribed by history; rather, they serve as a measure
of triumph, an index of the distance traveled in transcendence. The
male body suffers in these texts, but "real men" rise above it.

Perhaps the most significant recent shift in the national feeling for
the body, however, is something quite different: maybe it is less the
abstract ideal of citizenship that names the American in our era and
more the equally abstract structure of commonality called commodity
culture. AIDS places one outside the circuits of that culture, whether
that be those represented in gay publications like *The Advocate* or on
QVC. Pleasure and labor are both denied the body with AIDS.

I would like to close by thinking about the debate over political
correctness that erupted last year, and the reactionary position in that
debate that read gay studies as inimical to the national body. We can
read the canonical moment in gay studies as one part of an effort to
bust the traditional canon of American Studies; and (unlike African
American or women's writing in their anticanonical drives) it is not
just the list of texts we are interested in here—imagine American Studies without Whitman, James, Melville, Crane, Matthiessen, Santayana,
Hughes, Cullen, Locke, and the entire milieu of the Harlem Renaissance, or without women writers such as Cather, Stein, and Rich—
perhaps Jewett, and Dickinson. In other words, gay and lesbian writers
seem in some ways to be in the canon—just not as explicitly gay and
lesbian writers. What is beginning to shift is the way in which we read
these texts, and there are people who are quite upset about the legitimation of sexualized reading practices. Christopher Benfey, writing
in *The New Republic,* critiques Michael Moon, Eve Sedgwick, and
myself for being reductive in our interest in the sex lives of writers, not
really understanding that our interest is less in those lives than in the

ones that surround our own, that the question—for me at least—is how we read and how we use reading to negotiate social issues like sexuality. Benfey writes, "It's hard to see who benefits from having the poetry of Crane or Whitman, or the stories of Henry James, designated as simply and exclusively 'homosexual' in nature" (40); he misses the point here with his adverbs—no one imagines that homosexual writing is either simple or exclusive of anything. And certainly it is disingenuous to ask who benefits from this. But what is defended in protests like Benfey's are not just the names of hallowed dead men but an even more hallowed tradition of transmitting culture and ideological value through something called "literature," a cultural object he understands to be formed by aesthetic practices transcendent of embarrassing cultural or material specificities like sexuality (where "desire" is admissible, it can never take an articulated form: thus Crane may write about love but we should not "limit" that to questions about same-sex affection).

The question I would like to raise is this: what is the relation between homosexuality and the canonical, and why should gay studies appear as a threat to the national health? (This latter question will become more intelligible as we proceed.) Whatever our position within such debates, we are all familiar enough by now with the issues they raise to quickly sketch out a set of answers to the question, "what is at stake in the figure of 'canon'?" Ideological value, cultural centrality, what an earlier literary period identified as the centripetal force of culture; and in America, canon has always served the interests of nationalism as well. But there has recently been in the mainstream press a disturbing escalation of attacks on academics and their supposed wholesale jettisoning of Western values serious enough to warrant a renewal of attention to questions about literature and its value in American culture. The charge in such attacks is that this "fascism" or "McCarthyism of the left," as it is called, is more than an idle ivory-tower phenomenon; the movement toward multiculturalism and/or toward the punishment of hate speech on campus is represented as unhealthy for the nation and dangerous to its future (it is also interesting in this regard how issues around canon and hate speech are collapsed until it seems that democracy itself is founded on any student's right to wear, as one fraternity at Syracuse is now wearing, T-shirts that read [on the front] "homophobic and proud of it" and [on the back] "club faggots not seals"—the logo on this beauty is a rear end with a line through it stating "this is an exit not an entrance"). Obviously, reading William Dean Howells never caused such behavior in any group of people, but the defense of free expression is trotted out in such instances as the very thing the left has fought for and now wants to take away from others, and that issue is equated with a supposed left agenda wherein the canon would no longer be an educational force—disregarding the fact that the very notion of canon suggests there are distinctions to be made in evaluating language acts, that everyone's speech is not equal (so John Taylor's essay in *New York* can ridicule Catharine Stimpson for suggesting that Samuel Delaney's *Stars in My Pockets Like Grains of Sand* is just as valuable a read as Shakespeare, while defending the value of every voice in the student population, including racist, sexist, homophobic voices [see Taylor]).

There would seem to be a contradiction here. Although the analogy is seldom stated, these responses to recent academic politics imagine that multiculturalism is to America as AIDS is to the body: a foreign agent has invaded and if we do not practice "safer education" we will find a whole generation unable to defend itself from the opportunistic infections of the left. It is significant, of course, that the appearance of these pieces (in *Time, Newsweek, New York* [reprinted in *Reader's Digest*], and in columns by Kirkpatrick, Will, and others) has coincided with our adventure in the Persian Gulf, and we can read in that linkage how questions about literature and canon are sutured not only to national ideology but to the production and reproduction of bodies available for combat.[5] One of George Will's recent *Newsweek* columns makes this explicit by naming Lynne Cheney "secretary of domestic defense." This is Will:

> In this low-visibility, high-intensity war [in academia], Lynne Cheney is secretary of domestic defense. The foreign adversaries her husband, Dick, must keep at bay are less dangerous, in the long run, than the domestic forces with which she must deal. Those forces are fighting against the conservation of the common culture that is the nation's social cement. She, even more than a Supreme Court justice, deals with constitutional things. The real Constitution, which truly constitutes America, is the national mind as shaped by the intellectual legacy that gave rise to the Constitution and all the habits, mores, customs, and ideas that sustain it. (72)

We need to think of this as something more than the usual anti-intellectualism of the American press, and because the body finally is the site on which ideology is enacted, homosexuality (although it never appears in Will's piece) names for American culture a condition of intolerability not named even by the archfiend feminism or that father of lies, Afrocentrism.[6] Although these movements are also condemned in these attacks and are in their ways as threatening to the stability of American ideologies as is homosexuality, it is homosexuality that is always the flashpoint of common sense in these pieces, the moment when things have gotten out of hand. This has something to do with the fear of conversion and contagion, something not attached to feminism and Afrocentrism in quite the same ways. In other words, you can't *make* someone female or African American, but you might *make* someone (haven't you always wanted to make our sons?) queer. (Our daughters are another story: it is precisely feminism that destroys them, not by making them female but by perverting how they read that: so identity is at stake in a different way in that discourse. Homosexuality is a threat to the healthy male body; feminism is merely false consciousness.) In any case, canon is employed in American culture to produce a healthy national ideology, and that has always been its most apparent function. From the beginning of anything we might identify as American literature, the presence of a literary canon has been imagined as an indicator of national cultural health and maturity, one of the final measuring sticks of America's intellectual and global coming of age. And the invisibility of same-sex desire has always been necessary to the maintenance of that canon and to the ideological maintenance it performs.

If the canon secures—among other things—an ideologically correct body, a healthy body, we might think of that body as the site of a certain reproduction. Nor by this do I only mean to indicate the reproduction of cultural value and ideology that we have come to equate with canonicity, for in the terms offered by recent critiques of multiculturalism, left discourse fails precisely because it can give birth to nothing of cultural worth; it has no fructifying essence and produces only an atmosphere in which individuals read themselves as victims of oppression. We turn again to Will:

> feminist literary criticism is presented as a political act, liberating women writers from the oppression of "patriarchal literary standards." [One wonders what feminism he reads.] Thus does criticism dovetail with the political agenda of victimology. The agenda is the proliferation of groups nursing grievances and de-

manding entitlements. The multiplication of grievances is (if radicals will pardon the expression) the core curriculum of universities that are transformed into political instruments. That curriculum aims at delegitimizing Western civilization by discrediting the books and ideas that gave birth to it. (72)

Finally, the value of "proper" American values, so defined by George Bush and by the nervous academic right, is that they give birth, and they give birth to what? American values: in one of the great tautologies, to be "American" is to be generative of the American, to be (in one of Emerson's tropes that comes back to haunt us in the Reagan-Bush era) the party of hope for whom the future is *an American future* (Will's language positions feminism as an unnatural abuse of nursing and giving birth). And as we all know, homosexuality is nongenerative. Nor should we underestimate the importance of this figure. Eve Sedgwick has remarked how her nonreproductivity as a woman allies her to an extent with gay men, both marked "odd" in America because barren (see Moon and Sedgwick). So we have: maturity, reproduction, health, all secured by the canonical; does this begin to sound like a heterosexually inflected discourse?

It is probably clear that the figure of reproduction clues us in to how heterosexuality is at stake in the canonical and in health, as well, if we imagine homosexuality's historical and current links to illness. But I would like to return for a moment to the notion of maturity to think how it names the heterosexual allegiances of the canonical, especially since maturity is so closely connected to the other two terms. Not only is maturity required for reproduction (and in some communities reproduction is the required sign of maturity) but the developmental narratives of psychology—whether pop or Freudian—equate mental and sexual health with maturity in ways that gay and lesbian people have historically had to challenge. We see this very clearly in the way Hart Crane's contemporaries responded to him: because it indicated arrested development and a truncation of personality, homosexuality could not be the wellspring of a truly mature (that is, canonical) cultural vision. And while considerable effort has been spent in the past fifty years to erase from homosexuality the stigma of personal and cultural immaturity that contributed to Crane's tragic demise and misassessment—and to any number of unknown and now historically unknowable humiliations and rejections for other people as well—it may be time to rethink homosexuality's claims to maturity, for "maturity" lands us right back in a fetishized valuation of identity. To be mature in our culture means to have reached a developmental point of self-possession, and power accrues to such moments. But perhaps the paradigm of non-adult sexuality—precisely in its ability to free us from the tyranny of acceptable social identity—is our most subversive stance. I think of this not only in terms offered by Freudo-Marxists or Deleuze and Guattari, but in gay and lesbian appropriations of the terms "boy" and "girl," in the consistent locus of youth as a point of reference in both formations. This is perhaps the final meaning of Ganymede: not as an object of desire but as a figure for it—so we are not speaking here "for" pedophilia but against developmental psychology and the power of its narrative norms to shape cultural expectations in the field of human sexuality.

And if we shift the term from maturity to majority, and then think about minority, we can put an interesting double valence into play, one that leads back again to the canonical. Borrowing from Deleuze and Guattari's book on Kafka, Louis Renza years ago claimed Sarah Orne Jewett's fiction as a political resistance to majority culture in the name of a geographical and gender regionalism (see Renza). My question here is what happens if we think of all gay and lesbian literature as minor in this sense. Certainly we can add to the list of gay and lesbian writers associable with Jewett two names whose work stands in interesting relation to region and minority: Henry James and Willa Cather. In both cases—as in Jewett's—there is a concerted effort to resist the official identities and responsibilities of the adult world. In the case of both women writers, they express their desire to live in a prepubescent moment (Jewett's stated preference is age nine; Cather's pre-teen and hence also pre-gendered to the extent that sex-gender asymmetry is a cornerstone of what Judith Butler has called "the regulatory fiction of heterosexual coherence" ["Gender Trouble" 338], and the imperatives of adult identity introduce penalties for breaches in that system unthinkable to adolescent girls fond of dressing as boys and insisting that their name is William rather than Willa). It may not be immediately apparent that Henry James's work explores minority and regionalism in terms congruent with Cather's or Jewett's, but certainly we have for some time read his fascination with children as both an escape from and a projection of the sexual demands of adult social relations; and it is wholly possible that what upsets traditional readers of James when they encounter Eve Sedgwick's "Beast in the Closet" is less the imputation of homosexuality as central to the master's desire than the shift that now places his work in the category of the "minor" and the particular rather than the major and the universal. In any case, we might begin to think gay and lesbian writers as "minor" in Renza's sense and also as minors, as those who choose not to codify their selves according to the official relations prescribed by the social text. This would allow us to read adolescence less as a state of being in a developmental narrative and more as a trope for the shifting and multiple allegiances of being. And it may help us to read AIDS, and other categories of difference we have only begun to consider, less as conditions that fail to achieve the normal, less as spots we can at best put up with and at worst ignore. It may—if we embrace pathology—allow us to read as if from an other side.

Notes

This essay was delivered as a paper at Columbia University, New York City, Jan. 1992. The notes in this essay were prepared with the help of Alys Weinbaum, Patrick Horrigan, and Mario DiGangi.

1   National Basketball Association star player Magic Johnson led the Los Angeles Lakers to five NBA victories and more recently served as captain for the U.S. Olympic team. In the fall of 1991 Johnson tested positive for the AIDS virus. His stardom coupled with his HIV status continues to be a hot topic in media discussions of AIDS. In contrast to Johnson, the rather "ordinary" young woman, Kimberley Bergalis, grabbed public attention by joining forces with the media in her campaign to make her illness as visible as possible. Having become infected with the virus after a visit to her dentist, this unlikely victim's body became a common spectacle.

2   See Rampersad; Julien's film *Looking for Langston* (1989); and Hemphill's work on Hughes and Julien in Hemphill 181–83 and 174–80, respectively.

3   See Sedgwick's discussion of intersecting identities in the introduction to *Epistemology of the Closet* 1–66.

4   *An Early Frost* was directed by John Erman (1985); *Longtime Companion* by Norman Renee (1990); and *Parting Glances* by Bill Sherwood (1986).

5   Note, for example, the repeated coincidence of articles on AIDS and AIDS research in the same issues of *Time* and *Newsweek* that devoted themselves to patriotic coverage of the war: *Newsweek,* "Saddam's Endgame" and "Grief Counseling for Colleagues of AIDS Victims" (7 Jan. 1991); *Newsweek,* "Desert Victory" and "A Tempest in the Test Tube" (18 Mar. 1991); *Newsweek,* "Saddam's Slaughter" and "AIDS: Grin and Bear It, a New Humor Magazine" (15 Apr. 1991); *Time,* "On the Fence" and "When the Doctor Gets

Infected" (14 Jan. 1991); *Time,* "The Fog of War" and "Delays that Can Cause Death" (4 Feb. 1991); and *Time,* "Back to the Bad Old Days" and "Bumbling Toward the Nobel" (20 May 1991).

6   The major contemporary proponent of the philosophy of Afrocentrism or Afrocentricity is Molefi Kete Asante, whose work seeks to find the distinctively African roots of African American experience in order to situate it as an extension of African history and culture. In this respect Afrocentrism is an explicit critique of how a Eurocentric vantage point in scholarship and culture persistently masquerades as a universal one. See Asante.

AIDS in America: Postmodern Governance, Identity, and Experience

Do justice, cost what it may.—Henry David Thoreau

In a much-cited essay, Neil Hertz notes how the explosion of academic publishing in recent years induces in the subject enjoined to "keep up" a vertigo that recalls Kant's category of the mathematical sublime: an overwhelming series of numbers and/or sheer magnitude of information defeats comprehension and induces an abysmal intellectual and epistemological encounter that we mark as the sublime (see Hertz). Anyone interested in AIDS must suffer from a similar vertigo: the number of books, essays, pamphlets, and articles, the kinds of information, issues, and events that occur are so overwhelming in sheer number as to defeat any attempt at comprehensive incorporation by one person; the ever-increasing number of written responses to the history of representation of the disease makes it impossible even to survey recent literature much less to comprehend the totality of discourse about HIV since its appearance as GRID in January 1982. In addition, the exponential increase in cases and costs plus rapidly changing medical research and protocols challenge the intention of any individual to do intellectual and/or ethical justice to the various realities of the illness. As Sarah Schulman said at the Spring 1990 OUT WRITE conference in San Francisco, the field of AIDS and HIV continues to be transformed so rapidly that those who write about it do so with the understanding that by the time their words appear in print, they will be largely obsolete. Inscribed since its appearance as profoundly unimaginable, as beyond the bounds of sense, the AIDS epidemic is almost literally unthinkable in its mathematical defeat of cognitive desire.

But already we have here begun to make sense of AIDS, even if only in noting how it defeats our usual academic practice of careful, inclusive analysis. And we have also here assumed AIDS as an ongoing event, as something that moves within a history that is only partially *its* history. The mathematical sublime thus quickly gives way in the case of AIDS to what we might call the historical sublime, for even more than the mathematical, the historical sublime marks reading—and our stake in it—as an activity framed equally by demand and defeat, as the ground on which we are condemned to negotiate the difference between that which can be comprehended by the capacities of the intellect and that which can only be apprehended as beyond, in excess, or pitted against such capacities.[1] AIDS, for instance, can be apprehended—on bodies, in friends, in news reports, in changing populations, behaviors, and rituals: we know that it is in some undeniable sense "real," whether its reality be outside or within us. But the frames of intelligibility that provide it with even a meager measure of comprehensibility are notoriously unstable. This is evident not only on the macropolitical level, where intense battles over the meaning of AIDS have accompanied every stage of research and treatment in the history of the disease, but also on the micropolitical level, down to the level of the everyday (as anyone touched by it will tell you, the quotidian meaning of AIDS seems to change almost as often as the virus itself replicates—in wildly varying, if never quite random patterns). The gap between the apprehension and the comprehension of the disease is thus an asymptotic space where allegory persistently finds itself at play and where the ongoing histories in which AIDS unfolds (variously comprised of the viral, the personal, the communal, the national, and the global) are referred to larger and more masterful or authoritative histories that guarantee interpretation of its meanings and restabilize (sometimes ironically) those values it places at risk.

Like the systemic depletion that allows AIDS to appear as a seemingly endless number of symptoms and thereby remain both the same as and different from itself, the material effects of AIDS deplete so many of our cultural assumptions about identity, justice, desire, and knowledge that it seems at times able to threaten the entire system of Western thought—that which maintains the health and immunity of our epistemology: the psychic presence of AIDS signifies a collapse of identity and difference that refuses to be abjected from the systems of self-knowledge. Susan Sontag has noted that AIDS has surpassed cancer as the stigmatized term *par excellence* of contemporary culture, but her contention that it has the "capacity to create spoiled identity" (16), to alter how we know ourselves, is remarkably tame. Because it provides only negative structures of identification, AIDS is most notable for its capacity to produce non-identity or internalized abjection. Unlike the collapse of subjectivity noted in narratives of postmodernism that celebrate the simulacrum of inscription or the break with an oppressive history of metaphysics, the finality marked as and by AIDS includes an undeniably literal death, a death so irretrievably literal that its figurality must be continually exposed *as figuration,* as cultural critics like Simon Watney, Jan Zita Grover, and Douglas Crimp have been doing for more than half a decade; *and* (to reverse the burden of literality and figurality) the finality of AIDS is so in-wrought with configurations of cultural anxiety and dread that its literality must also be continually addressed in strenuous, referential narratives of victimization, punishment, resistance, and healing.

But in addition to offering us a focal point for analysis of the social and political intricacies of signification, AIDS also focuses for us numerous questions central to the current vogue for academic research and writing on the question of sexual minority. Who is the subject "at risk" in discourse about AIDS, in the homophobias attached to those discourses? Certainly it is not only those infected with HIV, and certainly not all those are gay men. But of particular interest here are two phenomena not perhaps to have been expected at the beginning of the epidemic: the appearance of large numbers of lesbian activists and post-liberation-generation gay men and women on the front lines of AIDS work. Let us ponder first of all how the two terms "lesbian" and "gay," driven apart by rapidly accelerating differences in visibility and privilege marking them through the supposedly halcyon decade of the '70s, have been brought together in this discourse—and how they remain apart. Surely it is not some lesser gift of generosity or conscience essential to gay men that leads to the oft-repeated assertion that, were the gay medical crisis of the '80s a woman's health crisis gay men would not be working for the cause with the fervor or numbers with which lesbians have responded to the crisis of AIDS. There are two important factors here: first, lesbians—as women—are marked in our culture in such a way that their "difference" is inescapable; gay men, on the other hand, are marked different in a way that does not preclude their "passing" or their negotiation of many of the privileges of masculinity even if known to be gay. Thus, the heartening lesbian response to AIDS may be due in large part to a heightened politicization of lesbian subjectivity (historically and personally) *before* the appearance of AIDS. Moreover, in its unyielding equation of value with white, male-embodied masculinity, American culture imprints a double bind on those on its margins: gay people of color and lesbians, for instance, may well find themselves alienated from white gay male culture, but they may also recognize that their own political future and visibility are bound in complex and equivocal ways to the struggle of gay white men. The dialectic of that recognition does not often work the other way: gay white men are less likely to see their own political fortunes at stake in what happens for people of color or women. It remains to be seen whether the numbers of younger gay men and women who have joined the battle against AIDS will continue their political work. Certainly they, too, know people infected and dying, dead or at risk, but *as a generation* they could choose to avoid AIDS, to see it as the issue of an older generation of gay men. Yet they continue to see their own subjectivity and freedom implicated in this battle. They have been politicized under the banner of AIDS precisely because one of the vigorously recurring allegories grafted onto AIDS has been its use as a mechanism for policing same-sex desire. These younger activists rightly perceive that what is at stake in public responses to the disease—from confusing, obscurantist, and moralistic safe-sex recommendations to violent Congressional eruptions of homophobia tied cruelly to denials of public health—moves far beyond questions of public health. AIDS has provided a site for surveillance of the most private bodily practices, and where subjectivity is framed through sexual orientation and preference, such surveillance calls into question any complacent desire for a comfortable "private life" (now read as the inadequate goal of gay liberation).

The political and the personal are, of course, so densely written *as intertexts* in the more recent history of minority discourse that it would be wise to say that it is only for purposes of analysis that we

even begin to think of them separately here; AIDS is a late and agonizing—but by no means singular—moment of crisis for a culture bent on
maintaining the fiction that the personal is not in any way political.
When we return to the question of experience below, we will reforge
the personal and the political in a more dialectical practice of reading,
but let us begin with a consideration of how AIDS has been inscribed as
an issue in the public forum. Perhaps the most visible and incontest-
able site of such inscription (and for that reason the site of the most
vehement contestations) has been the apparatus of government, and
while AIDS has forced a confrontation with government on virtually all
levels, the apparatus of the nation-state seems most appropriate to our
discussion here, for from the beginning of the epidemic in the United
States the federal government has housed the broadest powers of identification and intervention, and has therefore been at the center of
debates about public response.[2] In fact, municipal and state govern-
ments, with varying but usually lesser powers in this regard, have
become the target of so much political work in part because of the
vacuum created by federal irresponsibility. The failure to use their
power (effectively) to intervene in the disease constitutes the continuing charge against all levels of government by AIDS activists, and Randy
Shilts's narrative of its history, *And the Band Played On,* is—for all its
faults—one of the most successful texts to date to document the co-
lossal magnitude of bureaucratic indifference and ineptitude up to
1985 (Shilts's history, and not that ineptitude or indifference, stops in
1985). Shilts's writing makes a convincing case for reading the early
history of AIDS as determined by a remarkable lack of concern, communication, and cooperation on many fronts, much of that from within
federal agencies and among organizations like the Centers for Disease
Control and the National Institutes of Health. As baffling, however,
was a similar lack of cooperation among nations working to isolate
agents and treatments; as Shilts writes the history of AIDS, it would
have followed a far different trajectory in a world not structured by
competitive national economies that had in turn spawned competitive
nationalistic communities and practices in supposedly transnational
areas such as scientific research (scientists in the United States and
France were unable—due largely, as Shilts tells it, to the vanity of
Robert Gallo at NIH—to share research during the crucial first years of
AIDS). In accounts such as this, the government is charged with criminal neglect of its people,[3] and the invocation of crime seems appropri-

ate given the liberal philosophy that has historically constructed the nation-state as protector of citizen's rights by law and citizen's property and health through institutional intervention.

The allegory of value framed by the politics of the nation-state is a modern one, of course, its roots in the liberal politics of the nineteenth century. But despite our current need for such a model of government and for the needs-determined allocations it continues to promise if not deliver, it is not clear that an institutional framework developed during the imperialist excursions of bourgeois Europe remains a salient paradigm for political organization and analysis in a moment of multinational or postmodern capitalism. Ronald Reagan's simulation of same notwithstanding, postmodern governance is not based in the political representation of subjects under the beneficent gaze of a paternal presence. Jean Baudrillard, for instance, suggests that "the political and the social seem inseparable to us, twin constellations, since at least the French Revolution, under the sign (determinant or not) of the economic," but that "for us today, this undoubtedly is true only of their decline" (15). For Baudrillard, the entire politics of representation has eventuated in the implosion of meaning and the rise of a silent majority that functions to deny the meanings of the social; the masses are no longer potentially revolutionary, in need/search of some adequate self-knowledge, empowerment, or representation. The masses are not some "term which serves as universal alibi for every discourse" (66); rather, they

> no longer belong to the order of representation. They don't express themselves, they are surveyed. They don't reflect upon themselves, they are tested. The referendum (and the media are a constant referendum of directed questions and answers) has been substituted for the political referent. Now polls, tests, the referendum, media are devices which no longer belong to a dimension of representation, but to one of simulation. They no longer have a referent in view, but a model. (20)

The only political energy not bent to the implosion or denial of meaning in our era in the West comes from what Baudrillard terms "microgroups," those social forces that do not move passively and with fascination in the face of spectacle but insist on resistance, on decoding and recoding messages, "contrasting the dominant code with their own particular sub-codes . . . [by] way of redirecting, of absorbing, of victoriously salvaging the material diffused by the dominant culture"

(42–43). The actions of "fringe" groups in response to the AIDS crisis, therefore—not only their seizure of signification, for instance, but their absolute insistence on it, their insistence on the political, social, collective, and individuated meaningfulness of AIDS—might be read as working against the annihilating but passive power of the silent majorities (ACT UP's first motto: "Silence = Death"). Baudrillard's critique also suggests that AIDS activism has not been co-opted into the great institutional machinery of culture that currently recodes sign value as use value (found in the society of spectacle and its explosion of semiosis) but instead insists upon forcing spectacle itself into political use—hence the resurrection of agit-prop, street theater, poster art, etcetera.[4]

Also crucial here, however, is our recognition of a tension in American political and institutional life between the nation-state as a political entity and "America" as a term that ceases to designate the state and signifies instead a Platonic ideal of social consensus, homogeneity, and historical transcendence. Hannah Arendt describes the nation-state as claiming "to be above all classes, completely independent of society and its particular interests, the true and only representative of the nation as a whole" (17), but the illusory quality of that claim has never become as broadly apparent in America as it has, for instance, in Europe, due in part to much stronger anti-state traditions and movements there. In fact, the term "America" functions with such slippery teleological power that all critique of the state's overinvested interests ends only by invoking a more originary value for the same term (thus Reagan was elected partly on a platform of appeal to end state domination, yet that appeal was framed as a return to "America").[5] In American political discourse, "America" and the nation-state are not synonymous, and while the slippage between the terms is ever conveniently manipulated, the mythic term virtually always takes precedence and value over the more material one; conservatives may thus not only ignore the need for the nation-state to respond to population groups not visible within "America" (predominantly gays and IV–drug users in the early years of the AIDS epidemic) but may even cast those needs as anti-American, as a danger *to* rather than *within* the state. In addition, we encounter in American political discourse a rather unbreakable convention that the materiality of history disappear before the myth that America represents the end of (Western) history, what Jean-Philippe Mathy has noted as "the paradigm of posthistorical experience" (272). Long before Francis Fukuyama's recent apologia for the triumph of democracy as the end of history (see Fukuyama), America was conceived as the achievement of a radical break with the European past and—in its claim to utopian fulfillment and modernity—with time itself. According to Mathy, "the American mission, because it is conceived in *moral* terms, is the exact opposite of realpolitik" and Americans evidence "an inability to think in historical terms" (273). Thus, Reagan's wax-museum performances could borrow indifferently from Jefferson, Lincoln, Roosevelt, or Kennedy, stripping their words of historical context and of any ideological difference from his own use of them, producing a spectacle that *invoked* American history only to collapse it into the supposed timelessness of America *as idea.* AIDS, on the other hand, is not intrinsically historical (unless we mean by history the appearance of that which moves within myths unable to contain it), but discourse on AIDS invariably invokes the notion of history: research suggests a "natural history" of the virus (ten-year-plus incubation periods); gay and lesbian rhetoric links the fight against AIDS to Stonewall and to the entire question of gay and lesbian history; PWA rhetoric states that the ethics of our historical moment will be judged by its response to AIDS; journalists and experts alike project "the next ten years" or rehearse the present and past in a narrative behind which always hovers a specter of apocalypse in which AIDS functions as the demonic counterpart to the beneficent "end of history" coded in myths of America. In *Borrowed Time,* his elegiac memoir of the deaths of his lover and other friends, Paul Monette suggests that AIDS is inherently historical for the individuals it effects: gay men, condemned according to Monette to seek their history in "mythic fragments, random as blocks of stone in [Greek] ruins" (22), find that "the magic circle" of health and denial they were "trying to stay within the borders of" during the early days of the AIDS epidemic was "only as real as the random past" (6). AIDS thus becomes a rhetorical or epistemological nightmare as well: history, personal and/or collective, which should reveal pattern, reveals only a deadly but determining arbitrariness.

The other tenacious public discourse around AIDS, and one that is inseparable from the practices of the nation-state, is framed as science. From my latest T-cell count to Robert Gallo's theft of viral agents from French cultures, we have understood AIDS not only as a political crisis but also as a mystery to be solved by the power of science (understood as a pure domain of human knowledge wherein "nature" progressively submits to the power of human intellection and technological advance). Part of what baffles about AIDS, of course, is its resistance *as an illness* to this scenario of empowered science, but I am more interested here in the morality or politics of science, and in the failure of scientific communities to respond more fully and quickly to the demands of the disease. We may develop a method for reading the medical fiasco of AIDS in terms also suggested by recent philosophy and theory, particularly by Lyotard's notion of postmodernism. In what has become something of a touchstone, Lyotard suggests that the grand religious, political, and economic narratives of the past on which were premised the knowledge and totality of culture have fractured in an era of information (hence, "the postmodern condition"); as a result, "the temporary contract [elsewhere, 'language game'] is in practice supplanting permanent institutions in the professional, emotional, sexual, cultural, family, and international domains" (Post-Modern Condition 66). As Mathy suggests in his comments on Lyotard, the major contention in *The Post-Modern Condition* is that "the proliferation of autonomous and heterogeneous universes of discourse and behavior separated, and protected, by incommensurable differences [is] the social and political counterpart to the generalized disbelief in . . . 'grand narratives' " (292).

Translating this to the question of AIDS, we find a true incommensurability of discursive universes: as disciplines, medical and scientific research have indeed become separate, autonomous realms of knowledge and power unprepared to meet the emergency social conditions of the AIDS epidemic. Perhaps more sharply, the discursive universe in which gay men move and operate—a universe of open and various sexualities and (now) a universe of political rage—seems completely foreign if not still perverse to the medical community, the media, and the "mainstream" Americans constructed by that media.[6] Most costly among these incommensurabilities, however, is that between the nation-state and the populations most decimated by AIDS: still a cornerstone of the official "grand narrative" of American political and social life, the Platonic ideal of a classless, homogeneous State named "America" is incongruous with gay culture and the medical crisis AIDS forced upon it. Hence, as is suggested by Shilts's comments on the government's virtually immediate response to two other dramatic health crises of the 1980s (toxic shock syndrome and the Tylenol tampering case), the deaths of thousands of homosexual men did not solicit *any* government response for so long in part because homosexual men were not recognized as constituents of the (now infamously phrased) "general population," and in part because homosexual men did not constitute a rights-group in the eyes of a nation-state determined to read its population according to nineteenth-century demographic categories such as geography, age, ethnicity, labor, and gender rather than by behavioral patterns such as anal intercourse and intravenous drug use—*and* concerned mostly to guarantee the "health" of consumer culture, the non-toxicity of purchasable goods. Thus, AIDS becomes a rather obvious site on which to interrogate the beneficence of that autonomy granted within the postmodern, and this is perhaps one way to think the shift in gay male political needs and strategies pre- and post-AIDS: autonomy is desirable except as crises arise wherein the incommensurability of one site of culture with another (minority culture with medical, political, and scientific establishments) is written along lines of power that effectively prevent one of the parties in the "temporary contract" from partaking in the formation of the language game that constructs their social and political relations. This is the imperative of groups like ACT UP: to shift the language game, to speak, demonstrate, and demand in ways that are seen as inappropriate to the game when that game erases them or excludes them from its continual reformulation.[7]

If up to now our analysis has focused on rather conventional public or political sites, we must acknowledge that politics is not limited to the apparatus of the nation-state and its official mythologies. Critics who have turned their attention to other ideological sites in culture—and there have been many, particularly in the realm of the media and its construction of AIDS—have sought to enable resistance through critique and counterdiscourse. Simon Watney, Cindy Patton, and Jan Zita Grover are exemplary among those who have treated AIDS itself as a symptom, producing strong ideological readings in which AIDS discourse is exposed as thick with political meaning.[8] Unlike the media, which has tended to mystify the disease (and to literally mystify it: continuing, for instance, to identify it as "mysterious" long after its epidemiological paths had been established) (see Kinsella 134–36), these writers seek to demystify both the disease itself and the apparatus through which the media produce their mythologies of AIDS. Watney, for instance, contrasts the notion of "AIDS in Africa" to "African AIDS," pointing out how racist, colonialist residues function in the latter designation to obscure "the specific characteristics of the different AIDS epidemics in these countries [of Africa], constructing them in a spurious unity . . . which is immediately denied any of the cultural, social, economic, and ethnic diversity . . . taken for granted in

Europe and North and South America" ("Missionary Positions" 90). In
his earlier, trenchant analysis of British homophobia and AIDS, *Policing Desire,* he had suggested not only how "a particular virus, one of
the simplest life forms on the planet, has been used by a wide variety of
groups to articulate a host of issues and concerns, consciously and
unconsciously" (9), but also that many of those concerns were tangen-
tial rather than central to questions of illness and public health. For
instance, homosexuality has been so insistently at issue in the discourse on AIDS, not because the disease occurs naturally as a result of
homosexual activity, but precisely because the structure and stability
of contemporary configurations of heterosexuality require the invisibility and interdiction of same-sex desire, while the fight against AIDS
historically required that the lives of those framed by such desire be
made both visible and legitimate.[9] Similar analyses of the ideological
invisibility of black and Latino cultures in America suggest that AIDS is
also spread by power imbalances between those communities and a
governmental structure not concerned with them in any instance and
therefore without the requisite knowledge and apparatuses for education and provision of services in this particular, severely costly instance (see Alonso and Koreck).

If such media analysis implies that some representational practice
adequate to the political, ethical, and semiotic demands of AIDS ought
to be found, this writing also opens a critique of the media as an industry, as a commodifier of spectacle and information rather than as a
facilitator of some more genuine or analytical understanding. Here, a
postmodern critic (Baudrillard) and a modern one (Walter Benjamin)
would agree that Western culture has reached the limit or the end of
representational practices as they have traditionally functioned in alliance with knowledge of the social.

Baudrillard reads the media as destroyer of social meanings and as
producer of information-as-spectacle, and Benjamin marks this distinction as one between information and experience. But at stake in
both analyses is history and the dialectic between the subject and
her/his culture. Baudrillard may consider the curious passivity of the
masses a sign of their denial of their own historicity, while Benjamin's
analysis is more clearly wagered on classical Marxian claims, but both
fundamentally mistrust what Horkheimer and Adorno termed "the
culture industry." Benjamin writes, "with the full control of the middle class, which has the press as one of its most important instruments
in fully developed capitalism, there emerges a [new] form of commu-

nication . . . information" (88). Baudrillardian speculation on the collapse of meaning would reject *any* appeal to the meaningfulness of internalized process as anachronistic; we will take up below Benjamin's complicated and peculiar use of the term "experience" as a signifier for collective, dialectical knowledge. For now, let us see that information is not so much for Benjamin a representation structured by false consciousness, and open therefore to ideology critique, as it is a mode of semiotic circulation directly opposed to the cultural and subjective valuation of experience expressed in the following:

> Man's inner concerns do not have their issueless private character by nature. They do so only when he is increasingly unable to assimilate the date of the world around him by way of experience. Newspapers constitute one of many evidences of such an inability. If it were the intention of the press to have the reader assimilate the information it supplies as part of his own experience, it would not achieve its purpose. But its intention is just the opposite, and it is achieved: to isolate what happens from the realm in which it could affect the experience of the reader. The principles of journalistic information (freshness of the news, brevity, comprehensibility, and, above all, lack of connection between the individual news items) contribute as much to this as does the make-up of the pages and the paper's style. . . . The replacement of the older narration by information, of information by sensation, reflects the increasing atrophy of experience. (158–59)

Each item, each piece of data refers only to itself; "news" is the reification and sale of event, and this becomes even more apparent when AIDS appears in contiguity to—and hence as the scandal of—a culture of celebrity (the "shame" that inverts its "fame"). The deaths of Rock Hudson, Liberace, Willi Smith, and Amanda Blake are reported for their tremendous salability, but no connection between these deaths and the more political or even medical "facts" of the disease are encouraged in the reportage itself.[10] One need not subscribe to a fully Marxian theory of history and culture to recognize that any reading practice failing to link supposedly autonomous events and universes of knowledge—scientific research, op-ed pieces, the visible deaths of stars and the invisible deaths of so many others, public demonstrations, treatment advances, hospital overcrowdings, insurance and legal issues—is condemned to a limited understanding, if not to a simple repetition or invocation of myth. Nor ought such issues remain isolated in a frame marked "AIDS": they take place and meaning in more inclusive allegories of value that determine when, how, and if they will signify at all.[11]

But how do we reconcile the fact that the genocide of AIDS continues to take shape in the United States both as deliberate public policy and more privately in the lives and on the bodies of millions of individuals, especially when the invocation of "individual," like Benjamin's appeal to "experience" or "inner concerns," would seem to many to operate within a discredited paradigm of subjectivity that locates meaning in interiority? More generally, what valence do we wish to assign subjectivity in our analysis of AIDS? Diana Fuss succinctly states in her inquiry into identity politics in gay and lesbian culture that "to the extent that identity always contains the specter of non-identity within it, the subject is always divided and identity is always purchased at the price of the exclusion of the Other, the repression or repudiation of non-identity" (*Essentially Speaking* 103). If identity is not only a fiction but a particularly fragile, chiasmatic, and contradictory fiction at that, what is the value—political, personal, or ontological—of that identity marked "person with AIDS"? Has the prostitute who identifies herself as such merely accepted a false coherency in her life, and is it possible to read the subject marked "person with AIDS" as coherent in any case? Is the man who denies that his HIV-positivity allies him somehow with "them" (those "people with 'full-blown' AIDS") both politically reprehensible *and* accurate in his sense that "person with AIDS" constitutes a distinct category of being?

Susan Sontag's *AIDS and Its Metaphors* provides one avenue into answering such questions, for it rightly suggests that one of the numerous differences between the constructions of meaning written onto AIDS and those written onto earlier epidemics in history inheres in the fact that unlike AIDS, which is persistently interpreted as a judgment on the individual for sin or excess, "Diseases, insofar as they acquired meaning [in the past], were collective calamities, and judgments on a community" (45). Myths of identity *have framed* the interpretation of AIDS, and it remains a disease that attaches—rightly or wrongly—to identities: gay, IV–drug user, African, hemophiliac, infant, transfusion patient (the "guilty" and "innocent" "victims" are labeled through some category of identity that promises—falsely—to explain their contraction of the disease). Because AIDS has been read so persistently within a paradigm of group and/or individual identity, one of the continuing tasks facing those who respond to it has been to insist on it as a collective calamity. But one of those tasks has also been—because "person with AIDS" would otherwise signify non-being in a culture founded in and devoted to myths of being—the validation of any individual or collective identity threatened by the illness with erasure. We must think AIDS not only as a public issue of ideology, apparatus, and representation but also *as it is internalized and expressed* by those infected and effected, and we must do this, not because disease is a matter of privacy nor because individual experience provides unmediated authority and knowledge, but because "AIDS" as a signifier lodges in deep subliminal zones of memory, loss, and (im)possibility, zones that in the end are among the most crucial sites on which disciplinarity is inscribed and therefore potentially disrupted. Only because experience is material, dialectical, and collective can a critic like Benjamin be concerned about its atrophy, and we can employ "experience" as a signifier to mark not private and interior knowledges but the intersection between such knowledges and the collective, public structures that frame them.

When we turn to the inscription of AIDS in the discourse of private or personal experience, we find a number of powerful literary texts in the genre of memoir and confession, and a number in the conventions of domestic and family-crisis drama that establish the "likeness" of AIDS to—and its difference from—other social problems. Not all of those texts offer a dialectical understanding of AIDS as experience. It would perhaps be useful here to say something about the work attached to the name "Louise Hay." Hay is only one in what we must call a boom industry (those providing spiritual solutions or guidance in the face of the radical alterity AIDS introduces into a life), but her name has come almost to signify that industry, and her work ranges from books and tapes to seminars (weekly group sessions, attended by hundreds in L.A., are called "Hayrides"). Hers is, indeed, a labor based in and seeking the "affirmation" of people with AIDS, and for some Hay's work is truly transformative. Clients are encouraged to work with a mirror, to talk to themselves, to release rather than express anger, to love themselves; gay men taught to hate themselves or people with AIDS who internalize shame due to their illness can achieve a more positive self-recognition in these practices (see Hay). But the most pragmatically compelling aspect of Hay's work is also its most troubling, for it slips rather precariously from psychoimmunology to something closer to moralistic nonsense. Moving from a relatively nonjudgmental inquiry into the role of representation or mental imaging in physical well-being to a completely interiorized discourse in which illness, death, and even exposure to the virus are read as the free, "deep" choice of the individual, Hay's discourse has been attacked for its implication that those who fall or remain ill are incapable of effectively loving themselves, and for its mystification of AIDS as a gift to the self necessary to some crucial spiritual healing (not surprisingly, one available in her practice). There is nothing intrinsically wrong, of course, with any private experience, nor with private experiences of AIDS. But AIDS has required a continual vigilance against secrecy, shame, and repression, the hallmarks of that same (perhaps bourgeois) privacy that polices homoerotic desire: in that respect, completely private responses—while probably inevitable—seem insufficient for understanding the full cultural significance of the disease. The emphasis in Hay's work finally falls on an improved narcissistic relation as a cornerstone of cosmic harmony, and such transformations as result from it remain wholly contained within the individual's psyche. In framing this empowerment of the individual, Hay relies on a model of identity where the self is relatively stable, identifiable, and whole, where one recovers through meditation and spiritual growth an originary plenitude. The valence of purity and integrity of self in her discourse is clearly based in an epistemological imperative to keep the self separate from its others, something Donna Haraway has noted as the burden of most immune system discourse (see Haraway). Hay is not alone in producing as a response to immune system disease a discourse where nothing foreign invades the self, but her work is open to a number of critiques. More recent theorists of gay and lesbian subjectivity, for instance, read the political subversiveness and radical marginality of gay and lesbian culture as the direct result of their situation outside the ordinary structures of patriarchal culture, including the structure of stable, transparent ego that would seem to be Hay's model of subjectivity. Unstable and psychically eccentric in ways interpretable as politically transgressive rather than pathological, the ego structured by same-sex desire in poststructuralist paradigms offers—in the words of Jonathan Dollimore—"the paradox of a marginality which is always interior to, or at least intimate with, the center" yet not itself centered, and therefore key to the development of "new strategies and conceptions of resistance" (37). Judith Butler claims that "the gendered body" itself is "performative" rather than substantive, with "no ontological status apart from the various acts which constitute its reality" (*Gender Trouble* 136). That body, for Butler, "is not a 'being,' but a variable boundary, a surface whose permeability is politically regulated" (138). While the subjectivity constructed by AIDS should not be equated to gay or lesbian subjectivity, the paradigm of marginality and regulation would seem more than accidentally appropriate.

What we encounter in the field of AIDS—and of only marginal concern to someone like Hay—is the political regulation of the body around what is encoded as *the* supremely private site of accommodation to discipline: death. In her refusal to read the collective dimension of AIDS as a death that is at least in part an act of political regulation, Hay would return us to what Edith Wyschogrod has termed the authenticity paradigm of death, the equation of a "good death" with moral value: "Nothing so palpably illustrates the refinement and self-control of a person as the fearless and noble management of his dying" (3), the classic example being Socrates, in whose soul "is writ small the class virtues of the well-ordered state" (4). Wyschogrod offers a postmodern paradigm of authentic death as well, one where authenticity eventuates not through rational transcendence of death as an event but through acknowledgment of that death already represented in objects, persons, time, and desire. In the incorporation of death into life (her example here is Rilke), "the reciprocal relation between the acceptance of death and the profundity of the person holds: we redeem experience, render ourselves worthy of it, and it of us, by living up to the death in it" (10). But "neither the older nor the newer version of the paradigm can any longer provide meaning," Wyschogrod claims; they have been superseded by more recent histories of genocide and nuclear holocaust, by the intentional construction of death-worlds where the mimetic relation between an individual and his/her death is broken and "the living are forced to exist as if already dead" (34). The meaning of the death-world for Wyschogrod turns on intention, and although it arises from a technological society, its most profound function is mythical: "The death-world is not the extreme expression of technological society itself, for what characterizes that society is its rationality, its divorce from mythic consciousness, its uprootedness from the life-world. Instead the death-world is an attempt to make whole the broken cosmos by an imaginative act of radical negation . . . by consigning to itself all that seems worthy of death" (28). Plague will not do for this analysis because it seems to belong to a life-world "of indeterminate horizons from which phenomena arise" (17), rather than to the deliberate annihilation of vast numbers of people; the Holocaust, on the other hand, will serve as an example, and the point for us is that AIDS shares more, finally, with genocide than with plague. Like the death-worlds Wyschogrod investigates, there is only one signified in AIDS: all signifiers point to "death," and do so not as a site of the validation of the life-world but as its negation. And as in the death-worlds, it is the power of others to inflict dying that continues to shape the history of AIDS: the benign neglect of government agencies makes the epidemic a passive-aggressive act on the part of rational society (the institutionalization of power as indifference). AIDS shares many of the features of that man-made mass death that destroys the authenticity paradigm, and it is the promise of metaphysical redemption, of a repair of that identity-confirming experience of death that "healers" like Hay hold forth to those people with AIDS who desire—among other things—a meaningful death.

But not all invocations of the "experience" of AIDS need turn on this repair of broken subjectivity—or need not frame such repair as the reconstruction of a free, rational, and ultimately singular psyche. In an essay entitled "At Risk in the Sublime: The Politics of Gender and Theory," Lee Edelman narrates his participation in the October 1987 Lesbian and Gay March on Washington, constructing it as his "nearest approach to an experience of the sublime" (the sublime, of course, can only ever *be* approached), claiming that "the multitudinous unity and the mathematical sublime produced by our seemingly incomprehensible mass served to reconstitute our identity in the face of all our devastations" (220–21). Noting, finally, that such reconstitution is "theoretically regressive" through the constitution of "a coherent locus of subjectivity under the suspect banner of unity, idealism, and empowerment," when in fact the gay and lesbian community is often "painfully incompatible" even with itself, Edelman nevertheless reads the march as a "powerful and progressive force within the politics of gender" (227). While AIDS does not appear in Edelman's essay as one of the "devastations" inflicted by "homophobic America" on its gay and lesbian community, it is there as an unspoken devastation, and Edelman's comments might be taken as a gloss on that other powerful experience of collective identification in recent years that does in fact address the question of AIDS: the AIDS memorial quilt.

Although numerous reports of the experience of viewing the quilt mark its complex and overwhelming demand on apprehension and comprehension as a sublime rupture eventuating in unity, the object under consideration in this case seems to successfully resist the last move of the sublime (reincorporation) precisely because the unity it allows and constructs, the identity it offers through its collective scope, remains outside all of our corporate structures of knowledge. As in evidentiary encounters with the Holocaust, AIDS in this concrete memorial induces a contemplation in which all systems of signification seem inadequate. Ultimately, of course, some repair overwrites this abysmal grief, but as an artifact the quilt continues to challenge our understanding, and any cognitive accommodation that is forthcoming remains marked as radically by difference as by identity. Even as *labor,* the quilt is in some profound way disturbing (handicraft in an era of consumer goods, and motivated neither by profit nor beauty; handicraft where the trace of labor and its social referent remain visible, where that is indeed what defines its value—an unreifiable practice; labor seeking to intervene in an appalling alienation and both out of a love and anguish encoded on the surface of the object). It would seem almost to fulfill some of the folkloric function of narrative as Walter Benjamin describes that in preindustrial culture. Produced anonymously yet binding the culture together, the telling of stories during group activities and labor brings the "soul, eye, and hand . . . into connection" (108) and constructs a communal reference system of knowledge and value in which experience becomes recognizable through collective frameworks and becomes therefore communicable *as experience,* rather than abbreviated or atrophied in a world of information and industrial alienation. It is only in structures such as the quilt or, to a greater or lesser extent, in any demonstration or performance—in the making of artifacts about AIDS—that the disease can become meaningful in a way that allows those affected and infected by it to secure it as an experience and not merely as information. It allows as well an affirmation of identity not fated to succumb to the traps of affirmative, bourgeois culture in its determination to seal that identity and those meanings in a world of alienation and death. Only in such artifacts may the collective experience of AIDS be encountered, and only in encountering that collective knowledge may the gay and lesbian community continue to become visible to itself as something quite other than the site *par excellence* of social atrophy and alienation.

Notes

1   See the exchange between Neil Hertz and Paul de Man at the end of de Man's "Conclusions: Walter Benjamin's 'Task of the Translator.' "

2   AIDS is not, of course, a disease that occurs only in the United States—and

its effects are far more devastating in non-metropolitan sites, whether that be the Ivory Coast, Brazil, or (within the metropole) Harlem. Nevertheless, my focus here is on how AIDS has inscribed itself in American culture. Similarly, AIDS is not a gay disease, but its history is so densely interwritten with the more recent history of gay culture that I take up both in this essay.

3   One of the more powerful visual pieces produced by ACT UP represents the trace left by a bloodied hand and the written text: "The government has blood on its hands."

4   Douglas Crimp has written about "the graphic response to AIDS" in "Art Acts Up." Also see the introduction to a book he cowrote with Adam Rolston entitled *AIDS Demo Graphics*.

5   For an analysis of the history and ideology of this practice see Bercovitch.

6   For superb analyses of the construction of media audiences through the negation of homosexual desire and representation see Leo; Watney, *Policing Desire: Pornography, AIDS and the Media*.

7   Thus, when ACT UP interrupted U.S. Secretary of Health and Human Services Louis Sullivan at the Sixth International AIDS Conference in San Francisco in June 1990, many felt their actions an "inappropriate" silencing of the speaker; the point in that intervention was multiple, but among the strong reasons for pursuing it was the continuing nonrepresentation of those most directly effected by the epidemic in the very apparatuses (such as that convention, such as the Department of Health and Human Services) supposedly designed to address their needs, and supposedly doing an admirable job in that. The "game" in this case had failed to include all of its players, and some of those players—the ones with less power in the situation—decided to halt the game.

8   Here again we are confronted by the mathematical sublime, this time making it impossible to indicate all of the excellent work done in this field. In addition to those writers discussed here, see Crimp, *AIDS: Cultural Analysis/Cultural Activism* for an introduction to some of the central issues.

9   Even though the media have aggressively sought to recolonize and commodify traditional Others in American culture (just as one may now sample endlessly from exotic cuisines and cultures in the marketplace), this cannot be accomplished for gay and lesbian people. As Yúdice suggests, "the mainstream media have launched a campaign to demarginalize, decolor [and] degender[, but] gays and lesbians, much harder to demarginalize, are either stigmatized as the 'sinful' AIDS-ridden Other or are left unrepresented" (221).

10   When Halston died in March 1990, for instance, *People* (9 Apr. 1990) made his death a cover story: "He put American fashion on the map. He dressed Jackie, Liz and Liza. He died last week of AIDS, a broken man." Although his business failure is the biographical referent of the last phrase, it

signifies redundantly as the "truth" of any AIDS story (AIDS = broken), and while the magazine contains a four-page spread entitled "Fashion—An Industry Dressed in Mourning" and references to Michael Bennett's death from AIDS on its book review pages, there is nothing in it to suggest how these deaths are linked, linked to other social and political questions— nothing, for instance, to link it to the story on George Bush's refusal of broccoli (nothing on his refusal to speak about AIDS) or the story on a woman basketball player at Wellesley who "escaped China's brutal crack- down." Much less is there any attempt to shape the reporting of the disease as more than a series of single deaths and private tragedies. This is not, of course, true in the non-mainstream—especially gay/lesbian—press.

11   The first weekly news magazine to put AIDS on its cover (*Newsweek,* 18 Apr. 1983) featured a tube of blood marked "Caution: KS/AIDS" below the graphic, "Epidemic: The Mysterious and Deadly Disease Called AIDS May Be the Public-Health Threat of the Century. How Did It Start? Can It Be Stopped?" Above this are two small headers for other stories: "Chal- lenger's Men Take a Space Walk" and "Russia's Spies Get the Boot." The final indifference to AIDS during the Reagan years cannot be separated from what were national priorities of the political right—increased milita- rism, a renewal of Cold War hostility with the Soviet Union, a flat denial of funding for domestic issues—and the *Newsweek* cover remains uncanny in its framing of AIDS by these other two stories.

Hope

I don't care about professional success now—my concern circulates around my physical health and my emotional well-being. But I cannot give myself permission to see that as enough, to imagine that my life may be more important than my work. Now it is the case, I think, that the emotional health of the subject depends to a great extent on its ability to imagine itself a productive member of some community. And right now the frustration I feel and the intermittent uselessness are directly connected to a lack of focus in my working life. Why can't I figure out something to do? Why am I so uninterested in intellectual stuff? I still have ideas, I still perform interpretations; but my attention is all riveted on myself. I can't seem to pull myself out of myself. I can't seem to find something to believe in, and that keeps me unable to commit to a project.

I have thought that AIDS, of course, would make a good project for me. But what? Reading AIDS films? Why bother; we all know about them. Maybe what I want to do is sexuality and the lyric. Perhaps it's Žižek and a critique of ideology's conception of its own knowledgeability (I can look at the bookshelf and invent endless numbers of projects). Or perhaps it's simply time to take care of personal business: to talk with family and friends about my AIDS, to work with students. Maybe it's not my future fame I need to invest in now.

So I could write things about O'Hara or Ashbery or even Freud, and do critiques of Sedgwick and Moon—but it doesn't come together into anything. Should I return to the modern? If what this profession is all about is the production of something we call knowledge, what kind of "legacy" do I wish to leave behind? I think there's nothing I have to say that others won't say perfectly well; the stuff of gay studies is launched and its success guaranteed—so at this point, what do we do with it? What do we want? To be able to extend the discourse, to talk about ourselves more and more?

When I wrote *Hart Crane and the Homosexual Text,* I was not trying simply to be trendy—and yet I tried very hard to be up-to-date and new about everything, so I suppose it was kind of trendy. But I was trying to say something that I thought had not been said, to produce a first step in a new direction.

It comes to me (from where?) that the only thing I can possibly write about at this point is AIDS: all of the writing about it has been ideology/culture critique—how does that work? The representations have been silly, sentimental, pernicious, etc. (Now that we are past the point that critique will drive everything we say, what will we say?) I had thought at one point of expanding the "Postmodern Governance" piece into chapters: science and government (their incommensurability with our discourses about disease); politics and ethics; identity (start with Wittgenstein and the tumor as normal, but then try to get somewhere with the question of erotics, too, and the centrality of the erotic to identity [in the Renaissance, syphilitic discourse is never the end of the self], and representation (especially movies and TV). Perhaps.

When I look back at the paragraph above, I don't like it. The question is: why would one do this? What's the point? There may be one, but it isn't at all clear what it is. And yet, the place to begin is with trying to make some kind of difference in the way things are discussed and perhaps that is to bring personal discourse and the politics of experience back into AIDS discourse and "the political" more generally. But that seems weak and self-motivated. There has to be something more important to write about. AIDS is the text at the center of the book—that word by itself.

How the Eye Is Caste: Robert Mapplethorpe
and the Limits of Controversy

In marking one of the limits of the sex-gender system, male homosexuality stabilizes and therefore helps naturalize an arbitrary and seemingly increasingly unstable set of technologies and disciplines that operate upon the late-twentieth-century American body. The legibility recently accorded gay male culture by American academics should not obscure the fact that in majority culture male homosexuality remains a focus for tremendous anxiety and for (often) brutal fantasies that center not only on sexual practices *per se* but also on the failure of that system to keep its abject Other in its place. That failure is related to another, perhaps more fundamental, anxiety registered in the terror produced by male homosexuality, one that indicates the role of visibility in cultural epistemology: one must know what homosexuality looks like in order to avoid its multiple contagions, including now the more literal contagion ignorantly equated with it, AIDS. But if the linkage of male homosexuality to the visible has operated as an epistemological aid, it has also assured that homosexuality—even in becoming visible to itself—might never be produced out of sight of the pornographic.

The insistence of that cultural anxiety helps to explain why more controversy is attached to the name "Mapplethorpe" in the discourses around the recent Helms amendment to restrict NEA funding than to the name "Serrano," and why Mapplethorpe's photos of nude men and leather sex have functioned so prominently in that debate. At stake is not the fate of Mapplethorpe's reputation as a photographer, which seems at this point to be fairly secure, nor even the supposed "freedom" of the NEA and NEH to sponsor controversial projects. What is at stake is the fate of male (and by extension, female) homosexuality as a newly visible and vocal force in American culture. The denial of NEA funding in the wake of the Corcoran Gallery's canceled exhibit of the Mapplethorpe and Serrano pieces is only the latest installment in a concerted effort to build a right-wing national consensus out of fears that play prominently on homophobia and more or less explicitly equate male homosexuality with a national security risk.[1] One of the reasons to insist on the legitimacy of Mapplethorpe's work is to intervene in that construction and the political agenda that frames it. A victorious Helmsian would deny funds for AIDS research and education, for lesbian and gay rights, and would mark any representation whatsoever of gay male or lesbian existence "pornographic." Given its open wording,[2] victory for the Helms-sponsored restrictions on NEA funding would outlaw not only more sexually explicit texts but even so innocuous an image as Mapplethorpe's *Embrace.*

It is pointless to speculate on how Mapplethorpe might have responded to the recent Congressional flap: for someone intent on forcing the previously unseen into visibility, Mapplethorpe's politics were peculiarly privatistic. But it is clear that he courted, if not throve on, controversy. In Dominick Dunne's *Vanity Fair* essay/interview (February 1989), which was written in sight of Mapplethorpe's death from AIDS in April, 1989, and at his instigation, it is clear that Mapplethorpe enjoyed his status as *enfant terrible:* shocking Upper East Side circles with his leather chic and savoring the rather toothsome irony of the Whitney Museum exhibiting photographs bent on shattering the taboos of even the most bored, sophisticated patrons. One self-portrait exhibited there, for instance, shows Mapplethorpe without pants on, bent over away from the camera and turned back toward it with a demonic grin or leer, a bullwhip issuing from his ass like a tail. It is among his rudest images. But if the current publicity surrounding his

name makes it difficult to read against this tendency, we must remember that Robert Mapplethorpe was not only a photographer of the
(homo)sexually graphic. His work can be broken down into three
broad areas of focus: nudes, objects such as flowers and sculpture, and
portraits. And in his best and most interesting work, the protocols of
all three intersect, collide, and inform one another. What marks his
more unconventional images most singularly, in fact, is how poised
and balanced they are as compositions, their supremely high finish as
aesthetic objects conflicting with their occasionally violent and often
camp content. It would seem, therefore, a measure of the obsessions of
our culture that Mapplethorpe can be made out to be a gay photographer *tout court,* as, in the words of Dominick Dunne, "a documen-
tarian" of "the era of dangerous sex . . . of the homoerotic life in the
1970s at its most excessive, resulting, possibly, in the very plague that
[killed] its recorder" (126).[3]

The NEA controversy requires some brief comment here on the rather
familiar parameters of debates about pornography, but the issue I wish
ultimately to address in this paper is how desire is mediated in Mapplethorpe's work (comparing it to that of Bruce Weber and others in
passing). In particular, I am interested in how race figures as a discourse of difference and therefore as an incitement to desire, especially in Mapplethorpe's photographs of black men in *Black Book*
(1986). The controversy that has greeted that practice suggests that
these photographs mark a limit, one not as often considered as the
limit marked by the pornographic, but perhaps a more important one
in the context of gay male culture: the limit of *caste.*

We cannot here settle the debates about pornography that, unlike
virtually any other political debates on representation, have the curious power of bringing together those who are on every other question
antagonistic toward one another (Jesse Helms and Andrea Dworkin,
for instance). But we can begin by noting that definitions of pornography shift with the contextual arrangements that call it forth as a mirror
of desire, an Imaginary, for some population. It makes common as well
as theoretical sense to assert that as a category pornography is particularly difficult to define since taxonomies shift radically according
to the subject it places in question. That subject, in academic analysis, has almost always been considered female; only a few men have
stepped into the fray. Briefly, the debate centers on how one reads the
deployment of desire in pornographic texts. For some feminist arguments, all representation is violent in that it is phallocentric; therefore,

what is commonly identified as pornography (*Hustler* magazine, for instance) is only the latest instance of a regime and is exceptional only in its overt display of violence against women.[4] For other arguments that also proclaim themselves feminist, pornography sets in motion possibilities for desire that allow women as well as men to experience themselves as desiring subjects: therefore, pleasure in texts such as *On Our Backs* (a lesbian publication with explicit sexual content, both visual and verbal) or female pleasure in "straight" pornography must be accounted for as something other than ideological misrecognition.[5] It seems impossible to deny the collusive relation between patriarchal oppression of women and the sexual technologies and ideological apparatuses that have framed women as objects of male sexual pleasure, including but not limited to pornography. For its feminist apologists, however, there is danger in condemning pornography as the spoilage of an otherwise wholesome sexual domain in which women and children would be free of sexuality defined only as male lust.

But however one might seek to settle this debate, it is not clear that pornography has had the same function for gay male culture, desire, and subjectivity as it has had for female culture, desire, and subjectivity. For gay male culture, pornography has historically served as a means to self-ratification through self-gratification (or at least through the acknowledgment if not the enactment of homoerotic desire); and the relation of these experiences to patriarchal privilege and pleasure is not univocal. The national lesbian and gay quarterly, *OUT/LOOK,* ran a retrospective of the work of Tom of Finland, a Los Angeles illustrator who, in the words of one admirer, "draws good horny porn" (Patrick 6) that, in the words of one detractor, presents "over-muscled, thick-necked, jut-jawed, small-brained idols of male domination" (Wolf 5). In the debate that ensued on the editorial pages of *OUT/LOOK,* it became clear that what one set of gay readers found a challenging exploration of sexuality others found a corrupt and uninterrogated equation of power with sexual attraction and desire: patriarchy in gay butch drag. The point to be taken from this, however, cannot simply be that one of these sets of readers is correct and the other incorrect, nor simply that there are differing responses to sexually explicit material all of which are legitimate and defensible. Rather, the problem to be addressed in this case is the relation between the phallus of male homosexual desire and the phallus of male heterosexual desire, where "phallus" indicates both the power of the Symbolic order and the sexual organ associable with its articulation. This would require a full theory of the status of male homosexual practices within patriarchal culture, the distinction between those practices and male homosexual desires, and a clear articulation of how such practices and desires differ (if and when they do) from male homosocial, heterosexual, patriarchal practices and desires: I am not here able to complete that investigation. Nevertheless, we should not assume that phallic pleasure in one economy is equivalent to phallic pleasure in the other: as if a phallus were a phallus were a phallus. Recent gay male culture has indeed appropriated masculinity as a representational strategy for its own self-empowerment, and that appropriation has been equivocal at best in its commitment to other political questions. But this masculinity, appropriated, no longer takes its meaning solely within the structure of heterosexual institutions and practices; it is wrenched into intertextuality with numerous homosexualities as well. Al Parker may signify in gay culture, but so do the radical fairies.

A recent exhibit by Doug Ischar, "Household Misappropriations," facilitates an analysis of the relation between male homosexuality and masculinity as it can be read in the articulation among "the heroic male image," patriarchal power, and gay male domesticity (a non-exotic contemporary homosexuality). Ischar seeks to lay "tenuous claim to the heroic male figure as both co-optable subject and *attainable* object of desire."[6] The exhibit juxtaposes small, colorized reproductions of World War II images of masculinity (from *Life* magazine and other, more official sources) to written texts by Barthes, Genet, Voloinov, and others—*and* to five photographs of a contemporary "gay" man cleaning his apartment, washing dishes, etcetera. Ischar asks: "How does the macho-styled Gay man collude with and 'cash in on' the oppressive dominant function of this sign by silently 'passing'? . . . [H]ow does the heroic male figure (and his Gay inhabitant/claimant) resonate within the context of a sometimes mundane domestic life?" What results in Ischar's text is a dialectical process in which the iconicity of masculine bodies is put into play and into question: the "domestic" space is filled not by a "feminine female" who is absent from the cartoonlike scenes of World War II male-bonding, but by a "Gay male" who has no trace of "the feminine" about him. There is no means (or it seems to me politically unproductive) to say exactly where this dialectic eventuates, for the exhibit suggests that our own readings are bound to be "misappropriations." But Ischar's work is apposite here in that it marks the ideological mobility of images of the masculine, and does, in fact, allow us to read how "the buddy in the bunk above . . .

replaced the marble god replica, the buddy in the bunk below, his furtive and abject worshiper." And it suggests how a sign originating in a repressive practice (military hierarchies) may be dislocated from its initial site and installed in one subversive to the system in which it took its original meaning. We might also consider pornography (however we define it) as a text to be mobilized to effects that can displace violence and phallocratic order; we might think of its images as less irresistible and more open to misappropriation.

Leo Bersani, in his contribution to the special issue of *October* on AIDS, argues that sexuality exceeds its inscription, and that one of the values of pornography is its ability to reveal the tendency of sexuality to "demean the seriousness of the efforts to redeem it" and to make sexuality culturally safe, limited, and knowable ("Is the Rectum" 222). This is certainly correct—*in one sense.* But Foucault is also correct *in one sense* to recast Herbert Marcuse and suggest that the stimulation of bodies is as much a means to their control as is the repression of them: sexual liberation is never sexual freedom. How is it that both of these arguments (one in support of a libertarian attitude toward sexuality, one that would question the politics of that reading) might sway the same subject, might persuade me of their truthfulness and their analytical usefulness? This contradiction marks more than some personal inability to resolve the issue. It marks as well the overdetermination of sexuality (if not the entire representational economy) at this moment in American culture. The meaning of any particular sexual act, representation, or subjectivity cannot be reduced to a single valence. This "truth" is itself a refusal of the premise that grounds Helms's search for a pure signifier (both "pure" of illicit content and "pure" in its ability to produce a single rather than a multiple or contested meaning). It is this naive desire for stable reading that allows the alliance in principle between Helms and anti-porn feminists.

Given Roland Barthes's interest in the erotic and in semiotic density, it is not surprising that discursive multiplicity figures crucially in his reading of Mapplethorpe. In *Camera Lucida,* Barthes writes that pornography is itself "homogeneous . . . completely constituted by the presentation of only one thing: sex"; "at most it amuses me (and even then, boredom quickly follows)" (41, 59). Mapplethorpe's work, on the other hand, represents for Barthes "erotic" photography that "takes the spectator outside its frame . . . as if the image launched desire beyond what it permits us to see: not only toward 'the rest' of the nakedness, not only towards a fantasy of a *praxis,* but toward the absolute excellence of a being, body and soul together" (59). It is not possible, of course, to locate these "functions" with any critical accuracy.[7] Indeed, what constitutes such "excellence" as Barthes seeks is exactly what is at issue for Helms, Dworkin, the admirer of Tom of Finland, or Mapplethorpe; what Barthes sees as the monological text of pornography others may read as multiply dense and textured. But his distinction between the pornographic and the erotic is part of his desire to escape the overdetermination of sexuality in contemporary Western culture. *Camera Lucida* ends with a plea for egress from the alienation and ennui Barthes reads in current sexual fantasies and practices:

> One of the marks of our world is perhaps this reversal: we live according to a generalized image-repertoire. Consider the United States, where everything is transformed into images: only images exist and are produced and are consumed. An extreme example: go into a New York porn shop; here you will not find vice, but only its *tableaux vivants* (from which Mapplethorpe has so lucidly derived certain of his photographs). . . . [L]et us abolish the images, let us save immediate Desire (desire without mediation). (118–19)

Walter Benjamin is perhaps the ghost that haunts Barthes in this writing's prophetic outrage against modernity, and the invocation of his name should alert us to the impossible nostalgia of the passage: there is no unmediated desire.[8] We experience sexual arousal only in the context of difference or mediation, and in hegemonic sexual culture, that mediation has been defined almost solely through the discourse of sexual difference and the corpus of visual codes, strategies, and injunctions that support the "naturalness" of that difference known as heterosexuality.

Interestingly, Mapplethorpe's work arises from a homosexual site at precisely that historical moment (the late '70s and '80s in New York) when gay male culture rejected the discourse of sexual difference and its parody of male/female roles as *the* paradigm most appropriate to it. In it difference is staged, at least in the pictures of black men, through the discourse of race (in his works on leather sex, difference is staged through power relations and as pain, excess, and/or the exotic). As such, Mapplethorpe's photographs of black men cannot escape the charge of racism, of a fetishistic interest in black men that objectifies them and denies them their subjectivity. But Mapplethorpe's work does not present a single or consistent view of black men's bodies, and

he has his defenders. Kay Larson, for one, has written that Mapplethorpe's work in *Black Book* and other related texts investigates "a
formerly taboo subject (for Caucasians, at least)—the sexuality of black
men." She continues:

> Mapplethorpe has been accused of racism in using black men as
> objects of titillation and arousal. Those arguments don't hold up
> in front of the pictures themselves. . . . Mapplethorpe's black men
> are the first, in my memory of photographic history, to be given
> full dignity and equal stature as sexual beings—more equal, per-
> haps, than Mapplethorpe's whites, who tend to be a little nerdy by
> comparison. The photographer obviously enjoys the flow of light
> eddying and rippling off polished dark bodies, just as he does the
> excitement of treading on a taboo (fear of black men). . . . By
> placing his black men on a pedestal, Mapplethorpe seems to be
> working overtime to violate white clichés. (16)

Larson is correct to note the paucity of black subjects in the history of
photographic portraiture and in the tradition of the nude. Indeed,
Mapplethorpe himself claimed that one of the attractions of these men
for him as photographic subjects was precisely the novelty or intervention it allowed him as a photographer. What strikes one about Larson's
apology, however, is how, in attempting to justify Mapplethorpe's
work as nonracist, it participates in racist discourse itself. When Larson suggests that white men are "nerdy" in comparison to black men,
she admits (without acknowledging) that Mapplethorpe's work repeats the cliché of the black sexual athlete; and her appeal to "light . . .
rippling off polished dark bodies" as a violation of white clichés seems
wholly unfounded. The very notion of bodies with a "polish" almost
literally objectifies them, making them ebony sculptures in a white
fantasy; and far from subverting white clichés, the discourse of reflec-
tivity (which produces white fascination with the black man's "shine")
is wholly contained within racist paradigms (see, for instance, *Charles
Bowman,* 1980). Finally, impotence (and therefore the phallic power
or threat black men present to white power) figures prominently in
Larson's prose: criticisms "don't hold up in front of the pictures themselves." The "natural" potency of the black man's body (unproblemat-
ically captured in the photograph for Larson) disarms, makes impo-
tent, any response other than awe: it naturalizes the discourse that
situates it as an object for the gaze.

Mapplethorpe does (sometimes literally) place his black male subjects on a pedestal, and it seems that his interest in many of the studies in *Black Book* is in the variability of the eroticized body rather than in the power of the photographic apparatus to fix men in its gaze. But if the overall effect of works such as *Black Book* is to grant "equal stature as sexual beings" to black men, that does not in itself guarantee the text as free of the history and discourse of racism. Larson's claim for the "dignity" of these men is problematic, for instance, since discourse about the "dignified black" is deeply and tiresomely embedded in racist ideology. More importantly, one must insist that the sexual field is not the most appropriate or transformative site in which to contest the inequality that results from racial oppression, since Western culture has always sexualized its racial Others (see Bhabha; Gilman). Perhaps the most troublesome aspect of this is how black men and sadomasochism come to signify as equivalently exotic in Mapplethorpe's work and in the commentaries it has occasioned. Both are made to signify taboos and the "darkness" of the sexual drive (particularly the homosexual drive). Race is thereby made legible as a sexual practice rather than as a social, economic, and cultural difference with a history of great cost for those marked by it as Other.

Kobena Mercer has crystallized much of this in his response to Mapplethorpe's photographs, suggesting that they "facilitate the public projection of certain sexual and racial fantasies about the black male body," reminding us that not all of those fantasies are overtly sexual, and demonstrating how Mapplethorpe's work removes the black male body "from the social, ideological and historical forces that have sedimented and moulded received meanings into its shape and appearance" (n. pag.). Mercer's comments are in response to a London exhibit and to the British issue of *Black Males*. But the title of Mapplethorpe's book is not the only thing changed in the British issue of these photos: the British issue also contains a preface by Edmund White whereas the American text is prefaced by Ntozake Shange.[9] Thus, the book is produced to signify more as a gay text in Britain and more as a raced text in America. Mercer intervenes in this setup, insisting that one read the racial discourse within the gay. His critique of the work is damning, and he seems correct to insist that Mapplethorpe's photos are only another instance of "objectifying black men's bodies into an aesthetic ideal invested with what the *white male* subject wants-to-see."

While his point is wholly different, one can also see in David Joselit's essay on Mapplethorpe an admission that these photographs merely repeat conventional, racist images:

> the sequencing of *Black Book* implies a violent eruption/erection
> of sexuality in a setting of middle-class composure. . . . The *Black
> Book* is not so much a collection of portraits as a series of conven-
> tional images, some specifically related to stereotypes of black
> men. . . . Not only do most of his models have well-developed
> physiques, but many unselfconsciously display large, semierect
> penises. The effect of their exposed sex is not truly pornographic,
> or even erotic; Mapplethorpe allows no sense of sexual play or
> arousal to interfere with our opportunity to *look.* . . . [T]hese exag-
> geratedly phallic men look out at the viewer—and at Mapple-
> thorpe—with an expression of sullen threat, of suppressed vio-
> lence. Far from inviting intimacy, they hold it at bay. (21)

In addition to suggesting his culture's clichés about black men, Joselit
seems here to express his own uninterrogated attitudes: we perhaps
have differing notions of what constitutes a semierect penis, but I
do not read this as a dominant effect in the text; as to their unself-
conscious display, one wonders why Joselit would expect black male
models in nude photographs to be embarrassed by their genitals, large
or small. More importantly, while the portrait of Roedel Middleton to
which he refers does in fact hold the viewer at bay, to claim that it
suggests "suppressed violence" is merely to suggest that any black face
that withholds intimacy is a potential threat to the white man's power
otherwise to know and place black men in the visual field.

Those who read Mapplethorpe's use of black models as ideologically innocent tend not to theorize photography as a discursive practice whose meanings are intertextual with other social texts and practices. As Allan Sekula suggests, "A photographic discourse is a system
with which the culture harnesses photographs to various representational tasks" (87). There is no photographic discourse in which the
image innocently reflects a natural referent (the dominant theory of
photography in the nineteenth century). Moreover, Sekula argues that
"the photograph, as it stands alone, presents merely the *possibility* of
meaning. Only by its embeddedness in a concrete discourse situation
can the photograph yield a clear semantic outcome" (91). If it is true
that Mapplethorpe's photographic practices cross a number of traditionally discrete boundaries, taking up the conventions of art photography, for instance, in order to present material that seemed (before
he did this) incommensurate with its interests, we should recognize
that they are not therefore free to produce some "original" effect com-

pletely independent of the discourse of race in the culture they spring from and address. As Victor Burgin has written in another context, "any 'mood' or 'feeling' these pictures might produce, as much as any overt 'message' they might be thought to transmit, depends not on something individual and mysterious but rather on our common knowledge of the typical representation of prevailing social facts and values: that is to say, on our knowledge of the way objects transmit and transform ideology, and the ways in which photographs in their turn transform these" (41). The bodies of black men, like all that occupies the camera's gaze, are, as Burgin puts it, "*already in use* in the production of meanings, and photography has no choice but to operate upon such meanings. There is, then, a 'pre-photographic' stage in the photographic production of meaning which must be accounted for" (47).

Man in Polyester Suit is perhaps the most outrageous and potentially offensive image in *Black Book;* virtually all those who comment on the canceled Corcoran exhibit single out this picture as one of the significant transgressive moments in it. Clearly, this photograph is not coded as a pornographic text; its appeal is cerebral rather than libidinal, soliciting contemplation of the intertextuality of sexual and racial fantasies and confronting its viewer with the "pre-photographic" stages of social meaning upon which it works. In notes to the ICA exhibit of Mapplethorpe's work, Janet Kardon has written that this photograph "catches the viewer in a binary pull: The action cannot be perceived unless the eye constantly darts in opposite directions as in a tennis match, or, in this instance, between the mundane polyester suit and what outrageously protrudes from its trousers. Lurking within the conception of such photographs is a cunning and urbane humorist, always ready to surprise and outwit his viewer" ("The Perfect Moment" 11). In *Camera Lucida,* Barthes also claims that Mapplethorpe "shifts his close-ups of genitalia from the pornographic to the erotic by photographing the fabric of underwear [or of the suit] at very close range: the photograph is no longer unary, since I am interested in the texture of the material" (42).

Both Kardon's and Barthes's readings may be accurate (although the metaphor of the tennis match seems ludicrous: one wonders what tennis she watches), but they are not complete accounts of the discourse of this text. Mercer insists that we read the dialectical relation between the aesthetic cleverness encoded here and the pre-photographic set of meanings ineradicably encoded in the image. The strength of his critique is difficult to deny: "the racism thus presupposed is denied and white-washed by the jokey irony. . . . Sex is [still] confirmed as the 'nature' of black men[,] as his cheap and tacky suit confirms his failure to accede to 'culture' . . . his camouflage fails to conceal the fact that he originates essentially, like his dick, from somewhere anterior to Civilisation" (n. pag.).

We will return to this image, and to the question of how it may subvert this strong coding, but I want for the moment to consider Joselit's comment that Mapplethorpe's photographs are not erotic or pornographic—that they are simply an opportunity to look. Nothing, of course, is simply an opportunity to look; the gaze is always deployed or manufactured according to cultural power and is never innocent of ideology. But Joselit is correct, I think, in claiming that Mapplethorpe's work differs from the erotic and the pornographic as these are conventionally coded. The subjects Mapplethorpe explores (nude men and women, sadomasochistic practices) may indeed provoke response to them as pornographic or erotic, but the codes he employs in making his photographs frame them in the codes of art photography. These different photographic practices, of course, are not discrete but intertextual with one another; nevertheless, the codes of the art photograph position the viewer, the artist, and his subject differently than do the codes of pornography and erotica. The cover of *Black Book,* for instance, offers a sense of the posed elegance and artificiality that photographic discourse is for Mapplethorpe.[10] Mapplethorpe himself has suggested that even his overt interest in sexual organs is not always and only what it seems: "when I've exhibited pictures, particularly at Robert Miller Gallery, I've tried to juxtapose a flower, then a picture of a cock, then a portrait, so that you could see they were all the same. I would just like people to be able to get the real meaning" (qtd. in Kardon, "Robert Mapplethorpe" 25). What he does not register in this is that difference is already inscribed in these objects, and that any sameness he can produce among them as a photographer is predicated on his erasure of their social, material difference and its meanings.

Because Mapplethorpe's work, and *Black Book* in particular, places its subjects sparsely and aesthetically—almost clinically—before the camera, there is little space for conventional sexual fantasy. In that respect, his photographs are quite different from those of Bruce Weber, the photographer known for the dramatic style of his Calvin Klein ads who has a specific market for his work in the gay community. In Weber's commercial photography, the body is commodified; rather than being erased, background or setting functions as a prop to fantasy. His recent book, *O Rio de Janeiro,* for instance, repeats clichés about desire for and as the exotic that cannot signify without a locale. The dynamic of the gaze on the cover, in which a man stares intently at a woman whose sultry gaze is directed at the viewer, is wholly in keeping with a naturalized sexual difference that places women before men's eyes, and it suggests how we are to think about looking in the book itself. What we find inside is a by-now familiar postmodern, consumerist practice of locating men as well as women before the gaze, one that is not particularly transgressive since it does little to unsettle the placement of the viewer. Weber's work speaks to sexual fantasy in quite conventional ways:[11] its appeal turns on commodification and the power of money to inform desire; its emphasis is entirely on pleasure. The setting in *Rio* is exotic, requiring both the leisure and the finances to travel; there clothing and other commodities frame and mediate the body throughout the book, producing images that might function indiscriminately as advertisement for various products: a watch, mousse, sheets, cigarettes, condoms. Clearly, one cannot separate the fetishism of commodities in this discourse from the commodification of sexual fantasy or from its fetishization: everything here stands in for something else, and there is no question of the social relations among people that produce the relations among these "things."

Fantasizing reaches its zenith in Weber's book in a section devoted to the jujitsu champion Rickson Gracie. In addition to a number of photos that display his graceful muscularity for the viewer, there is substantial written text about him, his personal history is presented to the reader (including a male genealogy), and there are photos of his family (especially of him and his son). All of this information facilitates fantasy about him as the perfect type of the desirable male and codes that type as impossible to determine outside the structures of patriarchy. Mapplethorpe's erotic photographs, on the other hand, deny our ability to step into them in this way: at their best, they problematize and do not merely pander to our fantasies.

In *Let Us Now Praise Famous Women,* a text she composed from photos taken by women working for the Farm Security Administration, Andrea Fisher suggests that Esther Bubley's work encodes woman's resistance to the fixing gaze of the photographic apparatus in a manner that will help us understand Mapplethorpe's work. In *Girl Sitting Alone in the Sea Grill,* we find a different reference to context than that found in Weber's text: there is a context in this image, but it is one that does not totalize itself as a version of the viewer's desire; it does not participate in raising the discourse of desire to the level of myth, as do the photographs in *Rio*. Both the arrival of her Other and the arrival of our gaze at its fixity of her, Fisher implies, are deferred; "she stares away, with the oblique unfocused gaze of her own fantasy. She sets in train a flow beyond the unified place of the Other. . . . One is constantly sliding off the image, an imminent arrival forever post-poned" (105). This is similar to the way in which the cover image of *Black Book* both solicits our gaze yet remains closed to it. This image of the parting veil or curtain may or may not be an allusion to Du Bois, and it may or may not be an allusion to Derrida, but the parting of the veil certainly signifies that a rending is a rendering. In this case, the rending of the screen that has kept black men invisible in American photographic texts promises a rendering of them, a finding of some "truth" about them. And yet the image speaks obliquely, for it is turned away from the viewer, contained and closed within itself (head bowed slightly), its symmetry as much an ironic refusal as a revelation.

Fisher makes Marjory Collins's *Sleeping in a Car on Sunday in Rock Creek Park* the centerpiece of her entire inquiry into women's photo-graphic practice in the FSA, finding it resistant and rich in a number of ways: "sleep evokes that other sight of dreaming. Though she may become the target of desire, she is also immersed within desires of her own. While sleep may leave her powerless in the waking world, her silent desire also suggests a different register of power. . . . Sightless through dreaming, she becomes not only object of a gaze but, at once, its obstacle" (108).[12] For Fisher, the photographs in *Let Us Now Praise Famous Women* encode female desire as a site of power through their refusal to define the subject/object relation of their own gazing, be it fantasy or dream, and we see a similar (although decontextualized and therefore perhaps "mythic") figure in Mapplethorpe's study of Rory Bernal from *Black Book*. What we are presented with here is the body as the site of pleasure, but also with the ultimate enigma of that pleasure. What is figured here is the body's capacity for loss within a somatic realm that the camera can only ever signify and never represent.[13]

In the end, the black man's body, as Mercer suggests is historically the case in Western cultures, is often made to signify "flesh" for Map-plethorpe, and nothing more. But *Black Book* seems in some ways to foresee and answer that charge. In the first untitled photo in the book, for instance—the first of five that pointedly are alone in not naming the model and in focusing only on the body and cock (not the face) of the men—the text encodes some awareness of its own fetishistic practice by referring to a racial history that includes lynching (for instance, *Untitled,* 1980). This photograph can't help but call to mind a historical regime in which black men were not only denied the power to look (and the cloth here closes the veil of the cover cruelly back over the face of the man) but were hanged and mutilated, often for fear of the very thing here exposed: the penis. The not-quite-supplicant hands raised in a gesture superfluous to the body's condition—this is not merely a brutal and dehumanizing photograph, one that reduces the black man to his genitals, but is one where such objectification is implicitly questioned. I do not find it helpful to call this a racist photograph; rather, I think we might see it as a photograph that addresses racism—particularly as that which has sited itself in the sighting of the black man's sexuality. *Man in Polyester Suit* follows immediately afterward in *Black Book,* and I think it possible (without in any way denying the validity and strength of Mercer's analysis) to suggest that the text at least in part anticipates the response that it has made the penis the only signifying thing about the black man. Although its contrast to the cover is interesting in this respect, the context of the book as a whole makes *Suit* read as more than a cerebral play on the difference between skin and cloth (Barthes's and Kardon's readings). It also seems to make it signify more richly than Mercer suggests. If the image presents a view of what whites are certain is true—that the black man's true weapon, his penis, lurks large and always just out of sight—its placement in the book encourages us to read that as an interrogated practice and not simply as a joke.

I want to close by considering an image by another white American man, Robert Frank. His photograph of a funeral in St. Helena, South Carolina, part of *The Americans,* encodes itself (even in the tilting frame) as an intrusion on the social scene of a rural black community. The photograph records a ritual that remains unknowable to the viewer; unlike the dead man, who remains open to the camera's gaze, the people in it turn away with nothing to say except that they know something the camera can never share. Nor do they speak to one another. There is, in the photo, a sense of the unspoken understandings that produce and maintain community in codes of dress and posture, of generation and death, and even in the sense of an exterior space and its dissolving light—none of which has been orchestrated by the photographer, none of which is under his power.[14] The contrast I am trying to point to here is similar to one between Lewis Hine and Alfred

Stieglitz as noted by Sekula: "the Hine discourse displays a manifest politics and only an implicit aesthetics, while the Stieglitz discourse displays a manifest aesthetics and only an implicit politics" (103). From this perspective, Mapplethorpe's work has an implicit politics and an explicit aesthetics, while Frank produces a rather overt political text through its aesthetics. By placing *Funeral—St. Helena, South Carolina* against other images of the social text of Cold War America, Frank not only encodes the social subjectivity of his black subjects, but also allows us to read it within the larger structure that articulates it.

The retrospective of Robert Mapplethorpe's work held in 1988–89 was entitled *The Perfect Moment,* and the search for "the perfect moment" will always have an aesthetic agenda that solicits the forgetting of concrete discursive situations. Mapplethorpe's work returns us not to politics but to the question of vision, to the photographer-as-artist, and to the clever balance in his work. Its very undecidability (is the text in excess of its racism? is that conscious or unconscious?) becomes the hallmark of its status as "art" and of its producer as artist. In an interview conducted for the retrospective, Mapplethorpe said, when asked why he sees no difference in his pictures according to their subject, how he can see a cock, a flower, and a portrait as all the same: "The same is that I'm seeing them; it's my eyes that are photographing them" (qtd. in Kardon, "Robert Mapplethorpe" 28). This implies, wrongly, that objects are free of ideological associations—that they have not performed other, "pre-photographic" cultural work; it implies, wrongly, that the photographer's vision is somehow itself outside of ideological contradiction; and it implies, wrongly, that it is that vision that produces the meaning of the discourse—that intention is the final authority.

A man who, at the end of his life, was charging $10,000 a sitting was no doubt invested in his own authority as an artist. But the caste system into which Robert Mapplethorpe was taken up has an unsettling effect in the *Vanity Fair* interview noted above. Dunne reports that Mapplethorpe "gave a large cocktail party at his studio to celebrate his forty-second birthday," and lists as among those in attendance Susan Sarandon, Sigourney Weaver, Gregory Hines, the Prince and Princess Michael of Greece, the Earl of Warwick, Bruce Mailman, who was a managerial partner in the St. Marks Baths until it closed, gallery owners, museum directors, and others (187). What one notes with a chill, though, is that when discussing AIDS in this interview, Mapplethorpe points out that half the men in *Black Book* are dead: "Most of the blacks don't have insurance and therefore can't afford AZT. They all died quickly, the blacks" (185). At least in the world as *Vanity Fair* represents it (and that was the world Mapplethorpe was part of at the end of his life), "the blacks" remain a generic category, signifiers not of a sameness among gay men but of a difference that cannot be overwritten. These men were Mapplethorpe's friends, and in this comment he does recognize how privilege was encoded in their interactions. But the apparatus of *Vanity Fair* takes the political edge off that recognition, subsuming the deaths of these (here) anonymous black men into the more spectacular aura of the famous photographer, his celebrity, and the controversial works he produced. One reads here with an anger and a sadness that are all too familiar how race (and AIDS, and race-and-AIDS) are made to function as a difference more exploited than explored. That distinction identifies the problem that will continue to haunt analysis of Mapplethorpe's work. For all of their occasional power and astonishing beauty, these images too often stage racial difference in order to insure their own status as controversial texts. And that staging seeks to bypass the social history that has made it both necessary and possible, limiting its interventions in the social construction of the erotic to a problematic aesthetic effect.

Notes

I wish to acknowledge Patrick Bellegarde-Smith, Michael Awkward, Lynne Joyrich, Steven Mailloux, and Kathleen Woodward for their responses to earlier drafts of this paper. I wish also to acknowledge my critical dialogue with Robyn Wiegman, whose work has helped me better to understand both the economy of visibility mentioned here and the intertextuality of racism and heterosexism (see her dissertation, "Negotiating the Masculine"). I want to thank her as well for first bringing Kobena Mercer's work on Mapplethorpe to my attention.

1   This is seen as well in the intertextual dance of national defense and male homosexuality with which the Bush administration tried to explain the *Iowa* explosion, an episode without peer in the recent annals of staged homophobia.

2   In late spring and early summer of 1989, controversy over erotic photographs by Robert Mapplethorpe and photos by Andreas Serrano considered obscene (particularly a series entitled "Piss Christ" in which Serrano photographed crucifixes suspended in containers of his own urine) led Washington D.C.'s Corcoran Gallery to cancel an exhibit of them in an effort to forestall loss of government funding for these and other projects.

Congress, led by Senator Jesse Helms (R-NC), instituted new, strict guidelines covering the content of work to be supported through the National Endowment for the Arts, and placed the gallery that had originally supported Serrano's work (in Helms's home state of North Carolina) on a five-year probationary period during which it is ineligible for receipt of NEA funding. The Helms amendment reads in part, "None of the funds authorized to be appropriated pursuant to this Act may be used to promote, disseminate, or produce—(1) obscene or indecent materials, including but not limited to depictions of sadomasochism, homo-eroticism, the exploitation of children, or individuals engaged in sex acts."

3   Some of the more noteworthy contributions by men have been Ellis; Bersani, "Is the Rectum a Grave?"; and Watney, *Policing Desire: Pornography, AIDS, and the Media.*

4   The classic positions here are outlined by Dworkin; and Griffin.

5   Pat Califa is the most notable proponent of lesbian S & M (see "Unraveling the Sexual Fringe: A Secret Side of Lesbian Sexuality" and "Feminism and Sadomasochism"). Other feminists, who maintain that pornography is meaningful only through its engagement with cultural fantasies more often than not shaped according to patriarchal structures of subjectivity and oppression, nevertheless contend that there is the possibility of subversion, contradiction, excess, and transformation in it for individual women not posited as a single, unitary, exploited Woman (see for example, Kaplan). Sydney Pokorny, writing in *Gay Community News,* makes a similar case for the lesbian value of the spectacle provided by Madonna and Sandra Bernhard: despite its commercialization, Pokorny finds in it the "heretofore forbidden pleasure of watching two unabashedly uninhibited girls being incredibly sexual with each other" (10).

6   Ischar, "Household Misappropriations," Spring 1989, Visual Studies Workshop, Rochester, New York; all quotations from exhibit.

7   Barthes's distinction between the studium (the public meaning of the text) and punctum (the private meaning of the text) fails to note the first lessons of his own earlier work in semiotic theory that "private" responses to texts operate by codes that are, when one analyzes them, as ideological and socially constructed as more overtly "public" responses.

8   Or this occurs only in the Imaginary relation between child and mother, a dyad that *Camera Lucida* explicitly mourns the loss of.

9   It is surprising to find Shange's prose in celebration of the strength and beauty of black men given the context of recent American journalistic confrontations between black women and black men over the questions raised by sexual politics. One is left to marvel at how Mapplethorpe's publishers foresaw the controversy of his work and sought to forestall it with this legitimating preface.

10   Although Mapplethorpe has dismissed the comparison, his work owes

something to Edward Weston in its concentration on structure and surface as ends in themselves separable from the histories traced in their production as image. But Mapplethorpe far more than Weston *poses* his work: where Weston's work poses as the investigation of a structure it finds in natural objects (even the surreal nudes work this way to a certain extent), Mapplethorpe's work foregrounds the photographer's role in constructing the text. We may read this as part of his gay cultural heritage and its privileging of the aesthete and artifice.

11 *Rio* is not perhaps specifically "gay" in its semiotics, although Brazil has certainly come to function as a privileged (fantasy) site for North American gay men. Weber's postcards (of sailors, hunky men dousing themselves with water, male models posed dramatically and sexually in all sorts of social settings) have become icons in the gay community. On the day I purchased *Rio* on South Street in Philadelphia, three male store clerks borrowed it from me in three successive stores in order to ooh and ah over its contents—particularly Rickson.

12 John Tagg has written of the nationalist agenda of the FSA staging of the Depression as a meaningful term deployed through iconographically stable and exchangeable images ("The Currency of the Photography"). One of the important functions of that work concerns the construction of a culturally specific concept of class; we might note that Fisher's written text does not (despite her inclusion of images by Dorothea Lange and others that fall within the paradigms of class set up by the FSA's official vision of America). Fisher finds in Bubley and Collins exemplary texts for the encoding of women's desire as a register of power other than that which operates in the male gaze, but she fails to analyze how the meanings set in motion by these photographs operate only within a white, middle-class realm. See also Kozol.

13 Mapplethorpe's discourse of the body in *Black Book* is one of the body as a site of consistent vigor, tone, and organic unity. As such, we find a completely different discourse of the body in Mapplethorpe's work than in that of Johns Coplans, who has recently exhibited large, irregular self-portraits of his own seventy-year-old body. What one sees in these images from and of Coplans are shocking defamiliarizations of how the body wears its history, what one writer has called its "vigorous ugliness" (Phillips [curator of photography at the San Francisco Museum of Art], "A Body of Work," on Johns Coplans, The Art Institute of Chicago, April 1989), its fat, its small scars and deformities. Unlike the Mapplethorpe practice of presenting smooth, organically centered (if not culturally central bodies) in his work, Coplans presents a fragmented body, one that is perceived—like the body we know as our own before the mirror organizes it—piecemeal, not in proportion even to itself.

14 Yet Frank's work is different, more self-consciously "aesthetic" and "polit-

ical" than that of Arthur P. Bedou, a black photographer working in Mississippi and Louisiana until mid-century. Bedou's work records black life at a time when it was otherwise invisible within hegemonic culture—a group of men playing croquet on the gulf coast: starched white shirts under palm trees; the cars assembled for a summer picnic seen from a nearby hill; a *Photographer in Center of a Large Crowd* of formally attired black men and women (c. 1910). And this "simple" recording of public events—which has, of course, its own aesthetics—becomes its politics when the work is exhibited as part of a traveling exhibit from the Schomburg Center for Research in Black Culture, New York Public Library, Deborah Willis, Curator (seen at The Milwaukee Art Museum when I delivered an earlier version of this essay at the Center for Twentieth Century Studies in April 1989). It is this latter point that Barthes seems not to understand in his comments on the James Van Der Zee portrait he includes in *Camera Lucida*. By making that family grouping an occasion for his own memorializing project, Barthes fails to see how the very existence of the Van Der Zee text is based in a cultural Otherness that makes his aunt's dreary life— and his own patrician writing—not some "secret meaning" or "engagement" but a politically superfluous, if not offensive, appropriation of the text.

The Burdens of One's Deeper Debts

Michael Awkward

For Chris and Athena

It is impossible, of course, to fully know, much less repay, the burdens of one's deeper debts.—Tom Yingling, *Hart Crane and the Homosexual Text*

But every memoir now is a kind of manifesto, as we piece together the tale of the tribe. Our stories have died with us long enough. We mean to leave behind some map, some key, for the gay and lesbian people who follow—that they may not drown in the lies, in the hate that pools and foams like pus on the carcass of America.—Paul Monette, *Becoming a Man*

During my family's annual trips to the Philadelphia area, one of the stops we frequently make is the cemetery in which my mother's body was buried in 1986. After my first, tearful visit, when my pain was still so raw "it had no bottom and it had no top," these blues journeys home have taken on a nameless sameness, a disconcerting monotony. Now, when my family returns to the car to give me a few moments alone with my mother's remains, I try to do what I know I am supposed to: to talk to her. But these monologues make me feel utterly self-conscious, as though I'm merely mouthing the words of a dated script, fulfilling my role as the dutiful son to a mother who joked often that her children would not remember her after she had passed.

The living move on. My heathen heart tells me that the dead rest, even when they are not wholly "disremembered and unaccounted for," even when the son or lover, daughter, sibling, or friend believes that the dearly beloved "could never be dead until she herself had finished feeling and thinking."[1] For those who have passed on, death arrests development, kills the process of identity formation. It is the living who change, move, transform their thinking, their attitudes, world views, often with the assistance of their sometimes misremembered recollections of the textualized dead. Continually, we re-make even the dearly departed, to whom we cling because of what we believe they can teach us about our unstable living.

No putative cultural war against great dead white male writers will ever lessen the firmness of their hold on our cultural imagination, in part because most of the best of them—Shakespeare, Donne, Milton, Keats, Wordsworth, Tennyson, as well as others—not only provide for us a window to the past, but eulogize passing in a manner that instructs how both to survive it and, in its wake, to transform ourselves and our worlds. For my friend, Tom Yingling, the figure who most obviously illuminated the past and the future was Hart Crane. For me, increasingly, it is my mother, or my construction of her. And Tom.

II

In the days and nights immediately after Tom died, I searched for two letters he wrote to me that I hoped would help me better cope with his passing, neither of which I've ever found. The first was written in December of 1986, during our first months out of graduate school and away from Penn, and after he'd learned of my mother's death. The second was written in December of 1991 after what had been the longest period of silence that had passed between us since I met him at Penn in 1980. It was painfully impersonal, an emotionally distanced reply to several messages I'd left on his answering machine over the course of two months and a letter I'd sent him a few weeks earlier. This second letter signaled to me that he intended to maintain that distance. I believed that, because he'd found and moved in with a new lover, he no longer had time for me, no longer needed me. So I, in turn, tried to withdraw emotionally. I fear nothing so much as being judged unworthy, unwanted, not sufficiently interesting, by those few people to whom I've opened my heart.

When our friend Diane urged me in November of 1991 to visit him in Syracuse during the upcoming semester I was to spend on a fellowship at Princeton, I resisted, responding: Syracuse is hardly closer to Princeton than it is to Ann Arbor. I fought the urge to contact him, even at an affluent university's expense. When I skimmed the table of contents of Diana Fuss's collection, *Inside/Out,* I failed to notice Tom's piece, "AIDS in America." Had I seen it, I would not have suspected that it was autobiographically motivated. No one told me that he was giving a lecture at Penn, our old stomping grounds, forty minutes away from Princeton. Because he had sworn the friends we had in common to secrecy—new secrets, his to share with whomever he wished, when he was ready—no one told me he was dying of AIDS until a few days after my family and I had driven back to Michigan, until he had almost died, until the Kaposi's sarcoma lesions had covered him, disfigured him, until he could no longer move his bloated body. I didn't know.

I'd misread the clues, missed the interpretive keys. Was out of the loop. What kind of reader was I? What manner of friend? Maybe he sensed I couldn't have been of as much help to him as he'd been after my mother died, that he'd have to comfort me again. Clearly, he knew that I'd read death—her death and his—intertextually. Maybe I was next on the list, the next difficult letter, the next anguished call. Maybe much further down. Surely, he'd grown sick of confessing. I know I loved him. That he loved me. But I don't know if I could have handled knowing. I like to think I could have, that I could have been a source of some . . . something. As he'd always helped me. As I'd tried to be to him, suspecting, all the while, that he needed me less than I did him. But I was still prone to crying uncontrollably because I missed my mother. Maybe I could not have handled knowing.

But he'd supported me. Recognized my worth and ignored—or helped me to confront—my weaknesses. Comforted me. Our Penn friend, Athena, who, with her husband, Chris, drove with me from Ann Arbor to Syracuse to say good-bye to Tom, called him a teddy bear. When my wife, Lauren, and I visited him in Syracuse, nearly two years earlier, three months after my oldest daughter was born, I hugged him. I'm sure I always hugged him. But he said, "Thank you." For a hug? Why? When Chris, Athena, and I were leaving him for the last time, in the care of, among others, Steve and Celeste, Penn friends who'd flown in from Berkeley, he was bloated, dying, but lucid, and I blew him a kiss. It was horrifying to see him suffer so, look so, but I loved him, owed him in the ways you owe people who've opened their minds and lives to you, an unrepayable debt. I have tried to repay it. Am trying now, here. I will continue to try, though, as Tom certainly knew, I will inevitably fail.

III

Rereading Tom's engaging analysis of Robert Mapplethorpe's controversial *Black Book,* particularly in the context of others of his uncollected and/or unpublished critical and more personal writings, I'm especially struck by two things: (1) the skillfulness of his navigation of the troubled waters connecting race, sexuality, and caste in America, and (2) the manner in which the specter of AIDS haunts the essay, troubling his efforts to rehabilitate Mapplethorpe from charges that his representations of black men were racist. I'd been aware of the navigational skills as early as 1989, when I heard him deliver an earlier version of the essay at the University of Wisconsin at Milwaukee's Conference on Twentieth Century Cultural Studies. But the impact of AIDS as a contagion—in the essay's conclusion and, obviously, so many other places—did not strike me as powerfully then as now, since it has killed my friend.

Tom's writings add significantly to debates about AIDS and its representation, and to our comprehension of the difficulty of speaking about difference in institutional settings and by way of discursive formations that work to stabilize its meanings. Tom's struggle with difference—including scholarship/autobiography; homo/heterosexuality; white/black; poor/affluent; canonical/non-canonical—is highlighted by the anthology's structurings and choices, and makes me acutely aware of our differences. These differences seem to matter more on paper, in what was and is our place in the geography of identity politics, than they did in person. Particularly because my point of entry into this text, his last words and testament, is his engagement with another white gay male's engagement of black male bodies.

What does it mean for me, a living heterosexual black male, to join my dead gay white friend's lovingly organized body, to be positioned in its folds, to enter the most provocative and representative of the remains of Tom's body? Notwithstanding my previous sentence's play on the notion of eroticization of difference—we all know that not all difference is erotic to all people—I am well aware that I can say nothing to de-solidify the very real boundaries between life and death so as to return Tom to the world of the living. Nor can I, in any fundamental way, remake myself. In fact, I don't believe that I can do much to clarify Tom's challenging engagement with Mapplethorpe's representations of difference. And I want to resist the urge to wallow in my grief or to allow my black male presence to serve merely to legitimize what was, finally, in the age of academic identity politics, a risky intellectual project—a gay white male's effort, in the face of a resounding critique of this celebrated white photographer's representations of his racism, to explore "how race figures as a discourse of difference and therefore an incitement to desire" (61; this volume). I want to try to do with it now what I did not do when Tom asked me to read this essay before he sent it off for publication: interrogate his analysis. Point out not merely its many strengths, but also its tensions, its self-difference. And, particularly because he's passed on, I want to envision ways in which to keep aspects of his ideas in circulation just at the point this essay stops, gives up, and when Tom moves on.

Ultimately, "How the Eye is Caste" says less to me about the photographer's or Tom's participation in an erotics of difference than it does about the limits of viewing even the most controversial of representations, including Mapplethorpe's indisputably transgressive images, as scrutinizable only in the context of a history of "ideological associations" or " 'pre-photographic' cultural work" (74; this volume). However unwittingly, such a perspective fixes their creators and objects in endless, Sisyphean struggles with rocks that perpetually roll back down the mountainside. Tom's reading is, without question, theoretically deft and, for the most part, daring, anticipating and disarming virtually all possible reservations about Mapplethorpe's achievements and, finally, his own. He disarms by giving credit to the perspectives of both the photographer and his harshest leftist critics, and then, ultimately, by positing that the photographer's achievement is ideologically limited because of autobiographical statements about "the blacks," AIDS and his own artistic vision. Tom tells us that, in response to inquiries about how, despite their apparent differences, he can view "a cock, a flower, and a portrait" as the same, Mapplethorpe replies, "The same is that I'm seeing them; it's my eyes that are photographing them" (74; this volume). Taking him to task, Tom suggests that Mapplethorpe views "the photographer's vision [as] somehow itself outside of ideological contradiction; and it implies, wrongly, that it is that vision that produces the meaning of the discourse—that intention is the final authority" (74; this volume).

By the end of his essay, Tom has moved far afield from his initial defense of his subject's representational choices because of a desire to "insist on the legitimacy of Mapplethorpe's work [in order] . . . to intervene in that [Helmsian] construction and the political agenda that frames it" (60; this volume). After situating "Mapplethorpe" as a valuable sign within his own political economy, and offering reasoned interrogations of the positions of some of the photographer's most persuasive leftist critics, Tom concludes that Mapplethorpe's "peculiarly privatistic" politics inspires photographic texts that fail adequately to attend to the contexts in which the meanings of blackness circulate. Emphasizing Mapplethorpe's *Vanity Fair* connections, his "authority" as a celebrated artist, and a class position that permits him to battle the contagion AIDS in ways that his poor black subjects cannot, "How the Eye is Caste" concludes with a withering critique of the photographer's representational failure:

> One reads here with an anger and a sadness that are all too familiar how race (and AIDS, and race-and-AIDS) are made to function as a difference more exploited than explored. That distinction identifies the problem that will continue to haunt analysis of Mapplethorpe's work. For all of their occasional power and astonishing beauty, these images too often stage racial difference in order to insure their own status as controversial texts. And that staging seeks to bypass the social history that has made it both necessary and possible, limiting its interventions in the social construction of the erotic to a problematic aesthetic effect. (75; this volume)

Tom argued that Mapplethorpe's photographs are not sufficiently historically contextualized, evince the artist's failure to acknowledge his own complicity in structures of dominance, and demonstrate that he wants not merely to explore racial and sexual myths, but to exploit them. Much of the significant work in American literary and cultural studies in the last quarter century foregrounds ideology and self-reflexivity, and Tom relied heavily on this mode of inquiry, which is both beneficial and costly to his essay's overall persuasiveness.

Clearly, artists ought to be mindful of the complicated social histories their works evoke, the discourses in which they participate. But to what end, ultimately? Now that we have identified heretofore repressed and marginalized social categories, loosed them onto a now generally more accommodating academic and "real" world, we are bound to codify their meanings, to define, to establish boundaries between being and non-being. The search for authority and authenticity commences, is never-ending, clashes with our increasingly firmly held belief that identities are constructed. But, temporarily at least, strategically at least, we need to be able to invest them with more positive significations than those who had suppressed them could fathom. Hence the authority of female experience. Hence the Black Aesthetic. Hence what Paul Monette describes in his self-described gay male "manifesto," *Becoming a Man,* as a "watershed," his "breakthrough to my queer self": the discovery that "gay might not just be about whom we slept with but a kind of sensibility, what survived of feeling after all the fears and evasions of the closet" (272).

How do we know when we are being sufficiently attentive to the historical meanings of nonhegemonic status? What are the standards that govern their deployment? Clearly, artists and theorists must walk a fine line between creation and commentary, between envisioning the future and trying, against all odds, because versions of the past are never any less susceptible to "ideological contradiction" than the objects and persons Mapplethorpe placed before his camera, to recite aspects of the story correctly. If Tom is correct that Mapplethorpe's "intention is [not] the final authority," what is? Who is? These questions lurk in the margins of Tom's prose, not explicitly asked, never explicitly addressed, but clearly, Mapplethorpe is not invested with determinative authority. And Tom doesn't claim to possess or seek that authority. But if anyone has it, according to this essay, however problematic Mapplethorpe's use of the term, it is "the blacks," not all of them, certainly, but some, somewhere, adequately informed about the history and culture with which the photographer's work resonates and does not do justice, according to Tom.

These are difficult, perhaps unanswerable questions, but ones I pose because they help to point out the tensions in Tom's essay and, I believe, of the institutional moment of self-reflexivity and identity politics that, as far as I know, may be fading fast. But, sometimes at least, I feel it is not fading fast enough. I've been publicly rebuked for mistaking the availability to me of texts and analytical strategies that constitute the body of black feminist work with an invitation to enter it, assess its strengths and limitations, perhaps even add something to its heady mix. On such occasions, people who don't know me feel empowered to characterize me: I am the invasive other, biologically programmed and culturally inclined to render hurtful judgments, hold poisonous attitudes, strive to weaken the already weakened body. The signifying possibilities of my words and work do not liberate me from the cultural contexts in which my body, my gender, my black-male-ness, are read. No matter what I say or do, I am marked, defined, stripped, as it were, of the value of my individual negotiations of those contexts and situated within an economy of gender and race where my place is known, and the outcome of my interests in the black feminist body understood as something to be prophylactically guarded against. Like the photographs in Mapplethorpe's *Black Book,* about which Tom speaks compellingly before he confronts the nightmare of Mapple-thorpe's autobiographical, "privatistic" politics, there are aspects of my profile that render me incapable of what some would view as pro-ductive address. I am, in such instances, a foil, a whipping boy, a sign of the degradation of the class of humanity whose male and racialized bodies link them with me.

My challenge as a scholar has been to find a means of speaking productively despite and to that skepticism, to learn what I can from it, and resist, as an act of self-defense, the urge to flaunt strategically my record of service to its causes, which, weighed against the doubtlessly significant moments when I have transgressed against its ideals, might make me a welcome ally. As much as I understand that some will inevitably consider my presence to be transgressive, and me no more capable of resisting phallocentric urges and impulses than Mapple-thorpe is—as Tom put it—to "escape the charge of racism, of a fetishis-tic interest in black men that objectifies them and denies them their subjectivity" (65; this volume), I struggle to escape representative black-male-ness. While, being human, at times I stumble and falter, I believe that this is no idle fantasy of mine, not a function of some urge toward disembodiment or disassociation. Rather, it reflects my belief that while any investigation—of people, places, or things burdened by a history of representation—must necessarily begin with a strategic placing of the object under scrutiny in the context of appropriate in-vestigative and/or social categories, our responsibility, if we are to take full advantage of the rips in the social and institutional fabrics that have allowed us some sunshine and a few points of entry, is to prob-lematize others' placements, others' acts of scrutiny, others' histories.

In addition to contextualizing representation, we must also strive to ensure that all meanings don't remain fixed, don't stagnate, don't stra-tegically exclude the needy and the worthy systematically. Like the theorists of the photographic image Tom cites, including Allan Sekula and Victor Burgin, I recognize the inescapability, in interpretive situations, of referentiality, of cultural situatedness and representativeness. But art is forward as well as backward thinking, and we must never forget that.

IV

During the process of writing our dissertations, Tom and I talked on several occasions about the difficulties and consequences of doing work that was viewed as transgressive. (He explored textual manifestations of Hart Crane's homosexuality, and its consequences; my own, less ambitious effort, sought to demonstrate twentieth-century black female intertextuality in the novel.) I eventually came to understand that the phrase from Zora Neale Hurston's *Their Eyes Were Watching God* that I'd used as an interpretive center of my study because it visualized the sorts of cooperative black female intra- and intertextual relations I was trying to describe—"my tongue is in my frien's mouf" (17)—was infused with undeniably homoerotic potentialities that, while muted to some degree in the interactions between Janie and her "kissin'-friend," Pheoby, are unleashed within the tradition I tried to sketch by Gloria Naylor's *The Women of Brewster Place* and Alice Walker's *The Color Purple.*[2] I didn't know how to deal with this issue, how to handle it, whether I could, in addition to striving to offer an extended, albeit limited, exemplification of the formulations on intertextuality offered by highly regarded black feminist scholars, insist that the trajectory of this image's movement through time and space was not toward an achievement of ideal heterosexual coupling. Rather, that movement was toward the laying on of female hands, tongues, and bodies. What could I, a twenty-five-year-old heterosexual male at the time, before the development of a full-blown and fully embodied queer theory and gay cultural studies, have done with that?

   Tom told me that it was okay that I not tackle this weighty subject, too, one that, frankly, I wasn't—perhaps still am not—prepared to handle. I didn't—don't—know enough about gay studies, perhaps, but even if I were to get up to speed, I'm not sure I'm the one who should have done that work. That exploration would not merely have followed the general directions of black feminist criticism, but would have foregrounded a black lesbianism that, in a controversial moment in the pioneering essay, "Toward a Black Feminist Criticism," Barbara

Smith posited was everywhere.[3] I stopped short because I sensed that this was a boundary I should not cross.

My intent here is not to rebuke Tom, but to place my story next to his story, to acknowledge that his limitations are my limitations, are all of our limitations, and will continue to be so until we discover a means of consolidating the gains of these transformative times without rigidifying the meanings of "black men," "black women," "gay white men," all other others, and even "dead white male writers." A part of me resists the certainties of Tom's critique of Mapplethorpe, because I recognize there are ways in which it makes me—makes us all—a slave to "ideological associations," which we have become increasingly willing to challenge, and resist, when they appear in cultural contexts that we have marked as our own. Perhaps, given the boldness of his confrontation of the complicated issues Mapplethorpe represents, expecting Tom to problematize history and de-authorize "the blacks" would have been expecting too much. (Very few scholars seemed capable of such negotiations in 1990.) But I can try to do so now, and must. Certainly, I saw aspects of black women's poetics that I could not explore wholeheartedly, but others can, and must.

In that way, I want to believe, Tom's essay, Tom's book, Tom's living remain, like love, what Hurston calls "uh movin' thing" that "takes its shape from de shore it meets, and it's different with every shore" (182). I certainly hope so. I hope that we can engage, learn from, disagree with, perhaps even completely reject, aspects of Tom's formulations. "We" are those who knew him well, those centrally concerned with issues his impressive body of work interrogates, and those for whom he is a tragic victim of the AIDS contagion. All of these categories of readers can and, perhaps, will keep his words and work alive. And they will discover, finally, that Tom was not only a brilliant man, a courageous scholar, but also—his sometimes understandably forlorn reflections notwithstanding—much loved, much respected, and he is much missed. As Robyn put it in the letter she wrote asking me to participate in this volume, Tom Yingling was a sweet man.

Notes

1   In this section, I quote lines from Toni Morrison's *Sula* (149) and *Beloved* (336); and Zora Neale Hurston's *Their Eyes Were Watching God* (286).
2   These thematics appear also, most interestingly, in Gayl Jones's *Corregidora*.
3   According to Smith, a good deal of contemporary black women's literature

is "lesbian" because the women in these texts are generally "positively portrayed and have pivotal relationships with one another." To help her make her point, Smith turns to *Sula,* which she argues "works as a lesbian novel not only because of the passionate friendship between Sula and Nel but because of Morrison's consistently critical stance toward the heterosexual institutions of male-female relationships, marriage, and the family" (175). On a number of occasions, Tom discussed with me his interest in writing an essay on the homoerotic elements of *Sula.*

Knowledge Effects

Sexual Preference/Cultural Reference:
The Predicament of Gay Culture Studies

Any theoretical attempt to divorce homosexuality either from masculinity or from the fate of sexuality in general has to be seen as contributing to the maintenance of a status quo in which specific forms of homosexual practice are denounced and pathologized.—Klaus Theweleit, *Male Fantasies*

Although the exact dialectical relations among these aspects of culture are seldom explored as carefully as they might be, cultural theorists seem currently to agree that the fate of what Judith Butler terms "the regulatory fiction of heterosexual coherence" ("Gender" 338)[1] has been and remains indissolubly fused to the fate of patriarchy, capital, and the master race. We have even witnessed in the late 1980s what we might call the canonical moment in lesbian and gay studies, that moment when it has arrived at an institutional and disciplinary presence and authority quite recently unthinkable. The Winter 1989 issue of the *Lesbian and Gay Studies Newsletter* puts it thus: "If lesbian and gay studies have been simmering in North America for decades, in the last few years they seem to have come to a boil" (3). The evidence for this is available in the subject matter of conferences, essays, books, and dissertations, in the founding of programs and centers—even, although minimally as yet, in advertisements for hiring. Routledge Press, which has succeeded in marketing itself as the foremost publisher of texts in cultural theory, is rumored to be planning a list entitled "The Gay '90s" for this century's gay and lesbian '90s. Materialist, sophisticated in its understanding of sign and text, brashly disrespectful at times yet often impeccably credentialed: the study of homosexuality has been, in the '80s, exemplary as an archaeological investigation initiated and carried forward under the banner of an oppositional politics, and the strength of that work already available in the field seems to guarantee that gay studies—like the study of other minority discourses and experiences—will become an inescapable part of the way in which we negotiate the texts of culture.

What is perhaps most heartening is the fact that it is no longer only the tenured who have the courage to engage in this research—and we should not fool ourselves: to be openly gay or lesbian in the academy, to be working on gay and lesbian literature and theory (despite what seems to be something of a revolution in manners), is still to find oneself all too often embattled, belittled, and un(der)employed. This growing encampment on the margin of the academy, making its forays into the center, is therefore to be acknowledged and applauded for its labor. Those not within the lesbian and gay community are not aware of how extremely hard-won even the slightest legal or social concession toward lesbian and gay rights is or how perilously fragile the gains of the past few years remain. In an era in which the virulent hatred of lesbians and gays may still be expressed sanctimoniously on the national airwaves as well as in the House and Senate, in an era in which much sponsorship of anti-gay-and-lesbian legislation is linked to an indifference or backlash to AIDS (and vice versa), in an era in which funding for exhibits, research, and grants may be denied under the statutes of the Helms amendment (no gay-identified man received an NEA grant for 1990)—in this historical moment, the emergence of a strong gay and lesbian discourse in the academy is crucial to those who seek some site from which to speak against the assumption to power of the political right.

However, the exact parameters that will accurately and ethically delimit a distinct branch of cultural studies to be known as lesbian and gay studies have yet to be determined. Unlike feminist inquiry, where certain theoretical paradigms have found it helpful to separate the subject from her sexuality, lesbian and gay studies would seem to be inescapably wrought upon a sexualized subject. That linkage, given the increased commodification of sexual activity in modern Western cultures more generally, might make us wary of overreading the ability of transgressive same-sex practices to reshape the fundamental structures of our culture.[2] As Fredric Jameson wrote almost a decade ago, "[T]he right to a specific pleasure, to a specific enjoyment of the potentialities of the material body—if it is not to remain only that, if it is to become genuinely political, if it is to evade the complacencies of hedonism—must always in one way or another also be able to stand as a figure for the transformation of social relations as a whole" (74). At this moment in its history, lesbian and gay studies must vigorously insist upon the specificity of those oppressions that inundate and define the desires of people of erotic minority, but it must also continue to address questions about its construction within "social relations as a whole." We cannot assume that sexuality is the most significant— much less the only—cultural fantasy through which meaning and subjectivity are produced and through which desires are framed, policed, and institutionalized; however, we must not for a moment cease to read as lesbian and gay subjects, to interrogate the assumptions about sexuality that frame the ideological imperatives we face and inhabit daily. If the first of these two injunctions is akin to gay heresy, the force of resistance generated by the second is in direct ratio to how seriously one takes the demand that we move our project beyond the identification of homosexuality and homophobia and toward more inclusive questions about cultural power and the various relations it frames. Sexuality does not exist prior to and apart from the ideological work it performs in containing and articulating struggles and contradictions that appear more immediately on "other" axes of cultural power and difference; the legacy of Foucault, which can help us to read not only the care but also the politics of the self as a struggle with competing discursive and historical claims, ought to free us from the reifying gesture that threatens to inundate any and all projects in identity politics. . . .

. . . What is forgotten in the drive to achieve institutional presence and in the privileging of male or female homosexuality as a distinct facet of human culture? How is the object of gay and lesbian studies to be constructed? Such questions arise from my reading of two recent texts, David E. Greenberg's *The Construction of Homosexuality* and *Displacing Homophobia*, a special issue of *South Atlantic Quarterly*, edited by Ronald Butters, John M. Clum, and Michael Moon.

Let us begin here by considering the titles of these texts and the question of the subject. Gay and lesbian studies, like much of post-structuralist academic discourse in the past decade, has found itself divided on how it understands the subject denominated as "gay" and "lesbian." Nor is this only a recent debate: the struggle over taxonomy has been real for homosexual men and women at least since sexology came to authority in the late nineteenth century. Current wisdom suggests that "homosexuals" are not a transhistorical kind of human being, appearing with only local variation in different historical moments and contexts; rather, such wisdom dictates that all sexual identities and practices are constructed by and within the materiality of culture in force at the moment of their appearance. In other words, homosexual desire and identity—like heterosexual desire and identity—could not be considered intrinsic to and constant in human beings, since any instantiation of them would be legible only as the product of specific historical conjunctures of force and production that bring the subject into being and visibility. This argument (which one sees prominently in feminist, postcolonial, and African American studies as well) is known as "constructionism," and those who reject it, favoring some theory of a constant homosexual nature, are known as "essentialists."[3] We will leave aside here any extended discussion of the usefulness of these various positions and the validity of their claims, for the debate can quickly become tiresome. But both of these texts have titles that refer to this debate—Greenberg's explicitly, *SAQ*'s more slyly.

The stated purpose of Greenberg's book is to understand the "changing sexual typologies and images of persons who engage in acts we classify as homosexual," to produce "a phenomenology of homosexuality" that will explain not only the forms that behavior has taken throughout the history of human culture but also the governing and dissenting attitudes toward it (3, 4). He seems to seek, that is, not an essential understanding of homosexuality but a culturally grounded reading of how its construction has changed across history. This would appear to be something in the vein of Foucault's series on the *History of Sexuality,* and Greenberg offers some interesting speculation on the role market-capitalism and bureaucratic organization have played in the articulation of homosexuality in Western cultures. But the effect of Greenberg's work is quite different from that of recent outstanding texts on sexuality and culture largely in debt to poststructuralist theory (see, for instance, Eve Kosofsky Sedgwick, D. A. Miller, Butler, Jeffrey Weeks). Greenberg's history (499 pages, beginning with speculation on paleolithic rituals of semen ingestion and continuing through gay liberation) reads at times like James Michener and too often like a rehearsal of facts: Greenberg does not have the habit of questioning the empirical (in fact, he rather weakly dismisses Foucault for his lack of a properly empirical method). Thus, his sociology is neither critical nor oppositional but descriptive, in thrall to a dream of panoptic truth that Foucault among others has disciplined us to suspect. In a late address to the question of methodology, Greenberg writes that he had hoped that in his work "individual idiosyncrasies [in cultural attitude toward homosexuality] would cancel out, like the random-error terms in a regression equation" (493), allowing truth to appear in an undifferentiated and unequivocal form—as if language could offer us these "facts." What Greenberg offers is a reference text rather than a speculative analysis of the history of homosexuality; although he argues that *attitudes* toward homosexuality are constructed in culture, Greenberg's work falls outside the parameters of the constructionist debate since he has no theory of how the *subject* is constructed except as a mirror of such attitudes. This mimetic theory of social articulation in which the construction of the subject is not necessarily questioned leads, finally, to a logic of essentialism despite the rhetoric of historical change in the text.

Displacing Homophobia, on the other hand, would appear to imply a nonessentialist understanding of homosexuality since its implied way of doing justice to the question of sexual minority is not through celebration of the homosexual (whatever that might be) but through displacement of the powers that operate on and against homosexuality. But in saying that, we can see how the title also signifies that it wishes to "displace homosexuality" *as the issue for gay studies.* But even this move away from a reified notion of homosexuality is perhaps insufficient. In *This Sex Which Is Not One,* Luce Irigaray writes that "in order for woman to reach the place where she takes pleasure as woman, a long detour by way of the analysis of the various systems of oppression brought to bear upon her is assuredly necessary" (31). Irigaray has been berated for a logic of essentialism herself, of course, but the point here is well taken and its parallel for gay studies important: to displace homophobia only, and not to read the interdiscursivity of homophobia with "the *various* systems of oppression brought to bear upon" those who are defined *through* homophobia, does not displace homosexuality at all—it remains all that one sees, the only question one can ask about. Homosexuality is thus allowed to take its meaning without fuller reference to those other cultural systems that frame all sexualities as meaningful sites of subjectivity and political struggle. In John Clum's reading of Tennessee Williams, for instance, there is no interest in how the institutional practices of theatrical representation and the ideological imperatives of the '50s force Williams into a realist mode where heterosexuality achieves an unbreakable, mythic stature: by concentrating only on what he calls homophobic discourse (which also mis-signifies, since he seems by the phrase to mean the production of oppressive homosexual stereotypes), Clum makes homophobia an instance of unfair representational practice that refers only to homosexuals and homosexuality. Similarly, Sedgwick's essay on Willa Cather, which reads briefly the "invidious need of a passionate young lesbian to place, and at a distance, the lurid, contagious scandal of male homosexuality" in Cather's denunciation of Wilde during his imprisonment (64), does not ask other questions linked to a fuller understanding of the cultural history available to us in the signifier "Willa Cather": how/why national romance, cultural difference, history, and archaeology become crucial questions for her as a lesbian writer; how her lesbianism might be read as intertextual with the overwhelming antimodernism of her writing (how, that is, the archaic element signals anxiety and sublimation in her text) compared to the modernist experimentations of Proust or James (or Stein, whom Sedgwick does not consider). Sedgwick's comparison of Cather's crossing into masculine, heterosexual fictions with Proust's crossings of sexuality and gender in his fictions elides crucial differences between these two writers, not the least of which centers in the sexual ideology of the well-made aesthetic object. To begin to trace such contiguous obligations (which Sedgwick has accomplished forcefully elsewhere) would be truly to begin to displace sexuality and the phobias attendant to it from some of their more obvious cultural labor, including their more obvious academic labor as instances of critical desublimation.

Displacing Homophobia does assemble, however, work by some of the more prominent scholars in the field: Sedgwick writing here on James, Proust, and Cather; Stephen Orgel on Renaissance theatrical practices; Joseph Boone on Lawrence Durrell; David Halperin on classical Athens; John Leo on television; Robert Caserio on law and fiction; Ed Cohen on the Wilde trial as/and scandal; Moon on Whitman. Much of what is here is first-rate, but I would like in particular to address the essays by Leo and Caserio, for they exemplify gay and lesbian study of American culture at its current best. Both frame their analyses of cultural texts by moving *across* boundaries such as the legal, the literary, the social, and the sexual; in other words, they read the construction of sexuality within discursive practices that are not limited to questions about the sexual, and they seem to have moved beyond the literary canon as their object of inquiry. Caserio's essay seems quite important for those working in the field of narrative theory, for it works within ideological narrative poetics but against the tendency of that discourse to suspect all textual production—even resistant reading—as an exercise inevitably recuperated by hegemonic powers. Although he wishes to maintain that resistance is possible within power structures, Caserio is appropriately skeptical about how that resistance might be shaped, and by placing his discussion of two contemporary fictions against the Supreme Court's *Bowers* v. *Hardwick* decision, he argues that the subject of discourse is not always caught within the networks and operations of power it seeks to resist. In his reading, the demand for privacy and the desire for parenting by gays and lesbians cannot signify only within paradigms structured by and for liberal, bourgeois culture precisely because these demands subvert the heterosexual privilege encoded and guaranteed in those paradigms. Leo's work on broadcast television and the commodification of patriarchal masculinity (including the heterologies of male homosexuality) reaches beyond the question of justice to or discourse about gays and inquires into the process through which postmodern "cultural artifacts . . . repeat efficiently, quickly, and easily a point of view with 'recognizable meaning,' a homogeneity culturally produced and sustained which devalues difference" (48). Thus, his essay points toward a more inclusive reading of televisual and other cultural discourses and toward a reading of homosexuality in its structural relation to other sites of cultural power.

Other essays here show this discursive range as well, and gay and lesbian studies at its most profound will no doubt continue to construct an object of inquiry beyond the narrower limits of literary criticism, but this remains at issue for the reader of *Displacing Homophobia,* for gay studies as it appears in this volume would seem an overwhelmingly male, white project confined mostly to questions about literary texts (as the above list of contributors demonstrates). Only Sedgwick (approximately half of whose essay analyzes two texts in which Cather's protagonist is male) and Caserio (who gives Marianne Hauser's *The Talking Room* equal time with Terry Andrews's *The Story of Harold*) address the issues of lesbianism, and the introduction by Ronald Butters does not even note or explain its more general absence from the text. The closest one comes to any consideration of "race" is in Boone's references to the orientalism evident in Flaubert and Durrell, and in the introduction, where Butters complains that *Webster's Ninth Collegiate Dictionary* identifies racist slurs as "usually offensive" and homophobic ones as only "often disparaging."[4] We understand Butters's point: "faggot" *is* always offensive. But in a text that seldom calls attention to how racism and homophobia are intertextual, such hairsplitting over the refusal to grant gays equal oppression with "the ethnically slurred" (4) seems problematic, especially since the essays here consistently demonstrate that Western culture has managed (if sometimes—as with Wilde—at considerable expense) to make a place for white male homosexual authors and their texts. . . .

Finally, a few words about AIDS, which, for better or worse, conditions political discourses in the gay male community today (and, to a certain extent, in the lesbian community as well) and so offers itself as the nonliterary side of inquiry par excellence. There is one essay in this volume on AIDS, and while it is brilliant, its outcome is disturbing. Lee Edelman suggests that "there is no available discourse on AIDS that is not itself diseased" (316), no way, that is, to produce antihomophobic discourse in response to the injunction, "Silence = Death" (the ACT UP logo). Insofar as all discourse refers only differentially to its object, Edelman is right to suggest that there could never be a "pure" discourse of antihomophobia, that all discourses including antihomophobic ones are constructed through suppression of those self-differences that survive discursive sublimation in the trace. Edelman argues that to prefer (homo- or heterosexually) is to privilege, and to privilege is always to confuse the figurality of language with the literality of a referent. This not only would allow us to deconstruct the category of hetero- or homosexual, but occurs even on the level of cellular inscription: "The virus endangers precisely because it produces a code, or speaks a language, that can usurp or substitute for the genetic discourse of certain cells in the human immune system. . . . Subsequent to the metonymy, the contiguous transmission, of infection, the virus establishes itself as part of the essence or essential material of the invaded cell through a version of metaphoric substitution" (314). The logic of Edelman's argument is airtight, disarming all who would prefer a more referential discourse on AIDS; it is immune, one might say, to critique. No doubt hearing this complaint in advance,

Edelman ends the essay with a disclaimer: "I am sufficiently susceptible to the gravity of the literal to feel uneasy, as a gay man, about producing a discourse in which the horrors experienced by my own community, along with other communities in America and abroad, become the material for intellectual arabesques that inscribe those horrors within the neutralizing conventions of literary criticism" (316). But AIDS is not reducible to a set of specular "horrors" (even when asked to assume its most "literal" form), as Edelman must know, and I feel uneasy about the fact that Edelman's claim to dis-ease is intended to cover the question of whether his writing has done justice to the disease. One understands that AIDS activism often argues with a philosophically naive urgency, that ACT UP volunteers are not always sophisticated literary theorists, but "discourse," as Edelman's confession seems to deploy the term, does not imply that language is simply a system of essentially neutral differential relations.[5] It signifies as well institutional practices and inscriptions of discipline and knowledge across the body down to the level of what Foucault (in a figure uncanny for AIDS work) called the capillary. It is on that level, in fact, that the injunction against silence, against passivity, is addressed: to interrupt the production of discourses and the sites on which power is articulated when those discourses and the apparatuses that frame and legitimate their "knowledge" do not do justice to those affected by the virus and its concomitant political urgencies.[6]

I do not mean here to cast aspersions on deconstruction or to ask that those who practice it cede their authority to write on what appear to be self-evidently "political" topics (although we ought to remember that deconstruction reads language as simultaneously undecidable *and imperative;* the referential, that is, cannot simply be bracketed), but Edelman's piece forces an encounter with the issue of what it means to do critical and theoretical justice to any aspect of the social text—including the broader possibilities of lesbian and gay studies as a site of critique and foreclosure. In "Discussions, or Phrasing 'after Auschwitz,' " Lyotard suggests that "justice is . . . always possible, albeit as prudence . . . the prudence to make or speak the linkage 'that suits' in a particular case" (26). What is "unsuitable" as justice in Auschwitz's infamous version of the law for Lyotard is the incommensurability of the command "Die, I decree it": no "we" can be constituted in that command. "Auschwitz" becomes then "this impossible phrase wherein the law is not known, wherein it cannot be just, wherein the command cannot obligate, wherein man loses what is proper to him, namely, his *we*" (16). Similarly, AIDS signifies an incommensurability that now figures the contemporary impossibilities of justice. As yet some "we" remains (although who constitutes that "we," how and why, remain frustratingly narrow for those clearly under its sign)—but in variations on a "final solution" (unfortunately never completely buried in public discussions of HIV) one often still encounters its erasure.[7] Who is addressed, written about and on in AIDS discourse are questions one must continue to address to do justice to this contemporary figure of injustice. There is not one thing, or one correct thing, to say about AIDS: on that Edelman is correct. Our discourse about it is produced within the history into which the virus and its effects have been introduced, and that history is multiple, contradictory, vertiginous. But what we see in Edelman's reading of the disease is how gay studies can turn its attention to "new" objects of study without sufficiently interrogating the methods it employs; to follow out the metaphors of HIV, it would make more political sense to let our discourse infect and recode the message in master discourses and knowledges (from fiction to sociology to deconstruction) rather than let this "new" thing be treated through "old" practices.

Newsweek magazine's March 1990 cover story on the future of gay America (with a brief inset on the lesbian community: men are active and diseased, women domestic) cleverly renamed homosexuality "the love that won't shut up," intimating just how far the politics of sexual minority has advanced since the Wilde trials. But if that advance has been increasingly dramatic, much remains to be accomplished in placing sexuality (homo-, hetero, bi-, and other variations) before us as the almost overwhelmingly meaningful cultural articulation it is. Is it apparatus, discourse, subjectivity, practice, materiality, performance, or collective fantasy? When is it oppressive, transgressive, revolutionary, repressed, commodified, in excess of signification? What, precisely, is "it"? or will "it" always defeat our dreams of critical precision? The continuing move to displace homophobia carries in it not only an advancement of knowledges in the academy but also an urgency of lived relations that cannot be subordinated ethically to the production of academic discourse. In the end, the relation between the body and the page, like the relation between sexual preference and cultural reference, can be neither supervened nor collapsed. It is in the tensions promised in that asymptotic relation that gay and lesbian academic work can stake its most powerful claims to cultural relevance.

Notes

1   Feminist theory generally has been better than gay-male theory at examin-
ing the frameworks through which the expected congruencies and desired
disruptions of sex-gender linkages are constructed. Butler's recent work
extends this inquiry in extremely interesting and important directions. Rejecting the linear substantialist reading that moves from biological sex to
cultural gender to desire, Butler proposes instead that "the gendered body
is performative . . . [in] that it has no ontological status apart from the
various acts which constitute its reality, and if that reality is fabricated as an
interior essence, that very interiority is a function of a decidedly public and
social discourse, the public recognition of fantasy through the surface politics of the body" ("Gender" 336). Thus, for Butler, all identification (and
her work is principally concerned with identifications through gendered
narratives) becomes impersonation: "[G]endered subjectivity [is] a history
of identifications, parts of which can be brought into play in given contexts and which, precisely because they encode the contingencies of personal history, do not always point back to an internal coherence of any
kind" (331). See also her *Gender Trouble: Feminism and the Subversion of
Identity.*
2   The recent visibility awarded Robert Mapplethorpe, and the ubiquitous
defense of his work by the gay press and by gay academics, offers a signal
instance of this: forced to respond to Mapplethorpe with legitimating gestures (and that seems to me undeniably necessary), gay culture simultaneously finds itself unable to address the phallocentric appeal of Mapplethorpe's work, its occasional debt to racist discourse, and American
culture's increasing tendency to address same-sex cultural practices only
through economies of the masculine.
3   For a more comprehensive discussion of these issues within feminism,
around race, and for gay and lesbian studies see Fuss's *Essentially Speaking.*
4   One could begin by listing names—Baldwin, Lorde, Delaney, the Smiths
(not only Barbara, but also Bessie), Thurman, Hughes, Rustin—or one might
address the ways in which the outcome of racial difference has written
itself into the AIDS pandemic (Other Countries: Black Gay Men Writing,
a collective from New York City, currently has in performance an extraordinary piece entitled *Acquired Visions* that reads both the positive and
negative intersections of race, homosexual desire, and AIDS in American
culture). One might begin the arduous task of reading the racism in gay
discourse (even where, as in some of Mapplethorpe's work, the black body
is "celebrated"), or the equally arduous task of explaining the multiple
obligations that produce homophobia in the African American community.
Black gay culture should neither be read as simply a constituent part of
some larger gay culture nor be completely subsumed within the paradigms

of African American cultural studies: although *some* progress seems to have been made in addressing the question of lesbianism, it is not clear that the political imperatives that shape the discourse of African American studies can accommodate the question of male homosexuality at this time.

5   Taking AIDS "literally" is not always to be naive about representationality: in psychoimmunological work, mental imaging is read as a discursive intervention, and thought becomes a medical and political practice (sometimes staying alive is a subversion of power); in the work of Jan Zita Grover, Simon Watney, and others, analysis of the discursivity of AIDS is among the best work in cultural studies one can find. The literal and the figural are not, that is, always confused, even in "referential" AIDS discourse; but the question of effect is not bracketed, either.

6   In Edelman's essay, a logic of triangulation grounds every rhetorical turn, moving from the ACT UP pink triangle to a set of $x = y$ equations that run through the piece ("Defense = Discourse"; "Discourse = Disease"; "Defense = Disease"). But there is another triangle announced in the subtitle: "Politics, Literary Theory, and AIDS," and if superimposed on these others, that triangle suggests that "literary theory" centers the entire essay; it becomes not one side of a triangle but the equals sign itself. Everything *is* literary theory for Edelman, and literary theory is a language game. That "intellectual arabesque" does not for me adequately accommodate the disease as a social text or those who participate—willingly and unwillingly—in it.

7   In February 1990, the lesbian and gay community in Syracuse, New York, was forced to mount a locally unprecedented and massive effort against county legislation that would have destroyed confidentiality of HIV testing. The effort seems at this juncture to have been successful, but during it one sponsor of the legislation was quoted as saying that people with AIDS, if put in jails, should not worry—since they were dying anyway. Given C. Everett Koop's prediction within the same time period that AIDS cases in rural communities in the '90s will exceed those in urban communities, and given the appalling lack of knowledge about AIDS in many of those communities, such "intellectual arabesques" as Edelman offers seem the luxury of one untouched by HIV issues in their more urgent and emergent sites.

AIDS, Confession, and Theory:
The Pedagogical Dilemma

Perhaps more than anyone else, Cindy Patton has laid out for us the issues of AIDS in the classroom. As she points out, working through AIDS texts can mean a sometimes disturbing if not violent confrontation with our students' assumptions about pornography (any representation of the male body can become for our straight male students a pornographic text: so reading Douglas Crimp's *AIDS Demo-Graphics* brought the response from one of my students that he didn't want to have to look at some guy's dick on the page), about anal desire (an absolutely foreign state of being), (homo)sexuality (again, an alien notion for many), and the different communities that have been differently effected by HIV/AIDS. But even more, as Patton suggests in *Inventing AIDS,* "Teaching about HIV/AIDS . . . means teaching *how* to understand, how to *read* and *interpret* both the facts that bombard us and the context of our own lives" (110). Of course, all good teaching does this, regardless of the topic, but a text like Simon Watney's *Policing Desire* insists upon the politics of all media production and reception, and so one can use it to provide an object lesson in practices of reading that move beyond the question of how AIDS alone might be catachrestically (mis)represented.

To use the phrasing of Ernesto Laclau and Chantel Mouffe in *Hegemony and Socialist Strategy,* we can begin to see how AIDS is articulated to other social questions, and to see how any subject in the social field is always the site of multiple political and epistemological struggles. These kinds of interventions in ignorance about the disease as it has become part of America's (and the world's) social text may take place in the classroom—and may be especially effective in classrooms where it is not supposed to appear, such as a twentieth-century literature survey—and in other institutional sites through teach-ins, guerrilla theater, committee work, etcetera. As such, AIDS discourse provides an exemplary moment for questioning how we parse "knowledge" in the academy: for instance, reading various popular media, scientific discourses, and political arguments against one another takes us across institutional boundaries and allows us to ask how knowledge effects are indeed produced in our culture—and who has input in such production.

But for me, by January 1992, this was no longer enough; I felt that the time had come to come out to my graduate seminar about having AIDS. The fall had presented occasional difficulties with canceled classes, there were numerous rumors about my health circulating among department members, and I wanted in some way to try to make the text of my AIDS, to actively participate in if not fully control the way it would be constructed and re-constructed in a department of fairly aggressive readers. And while to some the emphasis on *my* having AIDS may seem to have placed me at the center of a circus of discursive babble about myself and the disease, I in fact chose the confessional mode as a way out of the specular: if I spoke about this, I would no longer be merely the object of others' fantasies—or at least their fantasies would have to confront some of my own statements about having the disease. I hoped that my confession might elicit not just the sympathetic response of students and colleagues but some speculation about the material conditions of pedagogical instruction as well: how we align bodies in classrooms, the schedules according to which "learning" is expected to happen in the university, how "knowledge" is assumed to be a disembodied thing.

The dilemma I wish to pose is how one might do this without falling into the experience/confession trap (in this case, Silence really does seem to equal Death, yet the politics of beginning a paper with a confessional moment are also questionable: does this only play out the drama of my own narcissistic investment in my illness and death?). Of course, coming out with AIDS is a pedagogical act whenever and wherever it occurs, forcing those outside the communities most directly affected by AIDS to think about the pandemic in a way they otherwise would not. The goal here is to let students read my body so they might see treatment effects, etcetera, and to include them in my disease process so that AIDS isn't just an abstract injustice or horror, something that relegates it once again to the specular. But what does it mean to make the professor's body the text of class: has it always already been that? Is it, to put it bluntly, inappropriate?

What seems potentially most radical about this is not just concretizing students' sense that they are at risk—at least for knowing someone with AIDS, but that the subject of knowledge should assume a body at all, which may mean it is no longer eligible to be imagined as a subject-that-knows. In fact, the body may be the thing that subjectivity cannot (ac)count—especially the body in illness, since any identity is confirmed through structures that integrate the body into an ideal wholeness. AIDS is not, of course, synonymous with a disintegrating body, but that is the threat. Finally, my take on AIDS and pedagogy is that it moves us beyond the extremely important and useful issues of representation and into an encounter with the embodiment of knowledge and so with embodiment itself, something we have never been able to broach in American education. What I want to develop in this paper is a further sense of how AIDS infects the discourse of pedagogical relations, and especially in the question of how the body becomes a site of knowledge and not just an occasion for it, and why that matters.

Note

This paper abstract was accepted by David Román for a panel on "AIDS: Politics and Pedagogies in the University" for the 1992 MLA.

Fetishism, Identity, Politics

Toward the end of *The Predicament of Culture,* James Clifford poses questions he considers central to the current realignment of knowledge in the postmodern academy: "on what basis may human groups accurately (and we must also add morally) be distinguished?" and, quoting from Edward Said, "How does one *represent* other cultures? Is the notion of a distinct culture (or race, or religion, or civilization) a useful one?" (273, 274). These questions are crucial not only to how we think about those groups Clifford explicitly considers (those that Western ethnography has traditionally marked as "distinct" and "Other"), but also to how we think about largely metropolitan lesbians and gays as they continue to work toward a more effective visibility and disciplinarity within the academy and without it. The academic analysis of lesbians and gay men, like the population such study claims to address and represent, has begun to insist upon itself as a distinct facet of human culture, able to resist the marginalization that has tended to mark it only as the scandalous or pathological Other. It is no accident that lesbian and gay studies has become important in postmodern discourses by analogy to other "species" of difference like race, class, and gender; and while the exact dialectical relations among these aspects of culture are seldom explored as carefully as they might be, we seem currently in agreement that the fate of heterosexuality has been and remains indissolubly linked to the fate of patriarchy, capital, and the master race. But what is the value of claiming a specificity for lesbian and gay culture and identity, and can we really read that claim as self-fashioned?

We have been witness in the late 1980s to what we might call the canonical moment in lesbian and gay studies: conferences, papers, books, even our own incipient star system; all of this attests to our successful intrusion into academic business as usual, and we should be especially pleased with this given the ignorant virulence that characterizes discourses about homosexuality in our more public debates as a nation. But we must also remember that canonical moments are not the fruition of some natural cultural process; they do not innocently mirror some object that precedes the attention of their critical gaze, and we must say this despite the fact that in this case our discourse seems spurred by a "real" population of "real" gays and lesbians beginning to be visible in American society. But if we think of canonicity not just as the generation of a list of validated texts but as the politically inflected codification of fantasies about collective origin or identity, then we can see that *this* canonical moment, *this* fantasy (like all others) has a dual function. It allows something to be entertained that otherwise would remain illicit (reading Henry James and Robert Mapplethorpe together, for instance), but it also occurs only at the cost of some repression. Apposite here is F. O. Matthiessen's repression of homoeroticism in what many take to be the canonical moment of American studies. As Jonathan Arac has pointed out, in writing *American Renaissance* Matthiessen disciplined his response to Whitman so as to erase the very thing he signified in the correspondence between Matthiessen and his lover: the legitimation of homosexual love. (Matthiessen, like Hart Crane and other gay men of the American 1920s, lived a contradiction between homosexuality and male friendship that Whitman's text seems to have promised to solve for them.) Repression functioned in this case to make homosexuality invisible, but the episode should remind us that disciplinarity requires repression and that our own shaping of the discipline of gay and lesbian studies might no doubt find the structure of its insights coaxial with certain blindnesses.

It may seem strange to think about homosexuality in terms of what it represses: same-sex desire has functioned almost as synecdoche for the repressed in our culture (thus, people now "come out" about anything once held secret), and we sometimes imagine that freeing it, nothing remains unsaid. But that is not necessarily the case. As Michel Foucault suggests in *The History of Sexuality,* the historical irony of our discourse about sexuality may well be that we imagined our political liberation to be somehow dependent upon what we could say about sexual desire as the ground of our subjectivity. If we take Foucault's notion of power and knowledge seriously, we have to be fairly skeptical about the level of subversiveness we want to read into the recent appearance of gays and lesbians as self-defined people in Western culture (and we might add, I think, in democratic culture). In light of such a skepticism, how might we more critically read the disciplinary or canonical moment of lesbian and gay studies? If many of those who identify as lesbian or gay do so within discourses and practices marked by an access to power and hence are "visible" or acceptable only within politically centrist terms, what could possibly constitute the political transgressivity of studying same-sex desire in our culture? On the other hand, isn't the demand that we signify always as politically earnest exactly what Foucault has in mind to reject when he calls us the "other Victorians," those who are determined to make sexuality and pleasure answer to ethics?

To return to repression: is there anything displaced or forgotten in our move from margin to center? If we think not, we have invoked a strangely monolithic structure of collective homosexual self-awareness uncontaminated by any trace of difference from itself, and that seems theoretically untenable. If we think so, we need to ask how our construction of a field to be known as gay studies might be changed by our knowledge that material has been lost or repressed in the process of coming to recognize ourselves as a distinct and specific facet of contemporary culture. In Foucault's words,

> Sexuality must not be thought of as a kind of natural given which power tries to hold in check, or as an obscure domain which knowledge tries gradually to uncover [but] as the name that can be given to a historical construct . . . in which the stimulation of bodies, the intensification of pleasures, the incitement to discourse, the formation of special knowledges, the strengthening of controls and resistances, are linked to one another, in accordance with a few major strategies of knowledge and power. (105–6)

That is, our discourse and our being are not organic appearances but arise at the nexus of other forms of knowledge, power, and pleasure, and our analysis of homosexuality or homophobia needs always to inquire into this structural density.

Perhaps the most obvious place to begin this analysis is with the question of gender and the screen of equality implied in the term "lesbian and gay": as my own prose demonstrates, lesbian and gay studies slips all too easily and all too often into simply "gay studies," yet never into "lesbian studies." This asymmetry should concern us, for among other things it suggests that "our" canonical moment is itself gendered and that perhaps what we have witnessed is the canonical moment of gay studies but not the canonical moment of lesbian studies—that lesbian studies may, in fact, be more powerfully configured under the rubric of feminism than under any accommodations gay men will ever collectively and institutionally be able to make to it. We might also interrogate the moment of our appearance for its attention to the social text of race: Marlon Riggs, the creator of *Tongues Untied* (1989) and other videos about African American gay men, offered a plenary address at this year's gay, bisexual, and lesbian conference at Harvard, and there has been an increased interest recently in making visible the lives and texts of gay men of color, as there has historically been an interest in race in the discourse marked lesbian.

But when much of the political energy of the summer of 1989 was taken up with an absolutely necessary defense of Robert Mapplethorpe's work, the issue of Mapplethorpe's racial politics was forced into the background or brought us apologies for his photographs of black men on the grounds that he was making visible a certain kind of "beauty" taboo in American culture. In the need for solidarity in that encounter with Jesse Helms and the right, race within the gay community became a difference legible in terms that did not offer any sustained attention to current and historical fetishizations of black men according to their "difference." In that, an inassimilable debate has escaped the mainstream in relation to Mapplethorpe's work, one centered on the charge of its appropriation of the black man as an erotic fantasy for white consumers (Kobena Mercer and I have addressed this question). In the end, however, we need to decide about these images less whether they are or are not racist in some final or definitive way than how and why they present to us a discursive formation and representation of race that is difficult to acknowledge under the regime of desire that produced and reproduces them. In other words, we all know that there is racism within gay formations—the question is not "is it there?" but "why don't we seem able to address and change it?"

To have framed both of these issues in this way is already to mark them as issues for democratic inclusivity, as terms within a discourse where representation becomes the "answer" to political oppression, thinking that if we take everyone into account in our own discourse, or give everyone voice, we will have evaded any oppressive practice. This is the logic behind cultural studies paradigms of race/class/gender/sexuality/age/ability/etcetera. We can generate that list and live in that logic, but this has rapidly become the most pointless of academic exercises—pointless not because the systems of social intelligibility marked by these terms have ceased to be crucial in the articulation of political power and control, but because the regime of representation into which they most often lead us has its base in a logic of liberal pluralism that we have by now sufficient history and reason to mistrust. Identity politics has lately gotten a deservedly bad rap all around. Although she argues at times for its strategic effectiveness, Diana Fuss has generally dismissed identity politics for its essentialist assumptions in *Essentially Speaking;* and Judith Butler has discussed in *Gender Trouble* how feminism can no longer retain the category of a unified (and ultimately masculine) subject as the base of its intervention.

The same issues have to arise for gay and lesbian studies. There is no such thing as "the homosexual and his/her truth," and if we imagine that as the project of lesbian and gay studies, we have surrendered to a lie at the outset. What we perhaps need to think about here is fetishism, as that has been defined in psychoanalysis *not* as the overvaluation of some part-object but as the denial of lack. All identity is fetishistic in that it is structured on the denial of self-difference and absence; identity, that is, cannot occur except through fundamental (and generative) misrecognitions. In the case of gay identity, the constructed fiction and denial of lack at the heart of subjectivity occurs through recognition of the tropes and practices of sexuality, offering sex as a center for otherwise decentered being. This is perhaps doubly fetishistic since we understand desire itself to be decentering, to be driven by lack. Thus, the trajectory of gay identity politics may read as follows: first, we stabilize desire (itself a move of considerable cultural violence) and then we attach the self to that desire almost as effect to cause, creating a second-order violence of identification.

Identity politics is the reigning philosophy of the popular gay press, however, and that should not surprise us since that press exists only as it can identify and exploit a demographic market. In the debate in that press about Jonathan Demme's film *The Silence of the Lambs* (1991), we can begin to see some of the implications of this as a practice for generating critique. In that debate, I was struck by the fact that the "pro-gay" position called for an end to homophobic stereotypes and for more positive representations of homosexuality, and that this was done in a way that imagined that we know and agree on what those "positive" images might be. In other words, a charge about the mis-recognition of homosexuality is leveled against Demme by people who claim not to misrecognize but to "know" it and to be therefore fully able to speak as and for homosexuals. There are a number of problems here, not the least of which is that we have no idea what kind of homosex-uals will be considered representative in such discourse. Furthermore, if Bill, the serial killer in *The Silence of the Lambs,* who is explicitly identified as someone without a conventional sexual identity, as a man who only imagines himself transsexual because he would otherwise have no identity whatsoever (he is, if you will, Gilles Deleuze and Félix Guattari's deterritorialized or schizo being)—if he is considered an image dangerous to homosexuals (the claim is that this film will pro-mote gay bashing), then why is Divine—in all her cross-dressing glory, eating dog shit at the end of *Pink Flamingoes* (dir. John Waters, 1972)— considered an outrageous, humorous, and ultimately liberatory figure?

My point is not that we ought to find Bill a liberatory figure as well, but that there is a contradiction in demanding "positive" images from mainstream culture while simultaneously embracing the strange and unusual in our own cultural space. In other words, if we need to get rid of Demme's film on political grounds, do we also need to get rid of Divine, since homophobes could conceivably find her image confir-matory of themselves in their misrecognition of her? The very notion that someone could say—in the discourse of identity politics—what homosexuals do or do not, should or should not look, sound, and be like is a potentially dangerous trap we may not be able to escape from once we decide to enter it. Moreover, as theorists of desire from Sig-mund Freud and Georges Bataille to Leo Bersani have noted, sexuality seems always destined to be determined as much by misrecognition as by anything we might term an accurate cognition *and* to remain in ex-cess of any theoretical or political moves to enlist it in the service of cultural mobility. Sexuality is imbricated with violence and death in virtually all its manifestations, and to attempt to find or articulate a clean, acceptable desire—especially a homosexuality imagined in this way—should be nearly unthinkable. If we are to build a critique of culture and an active alternative community based in the rejection of those terms and practices that have heretofore constituted the disciplinary or canonical formation of desire along unswervingly heterosexual lines, we must strenuously reject the wisdom of institutionalizing a counterdiscipline or alternative list of acceptable and unacceptable sexualities.

This would seem to be the impetus behind the new politically fashionable use of the term "queer" to designate things nonheterosexual— as in Queer Nation or what a cover of *The Advocate,* referring to *Poison* and *Paris Is Burning,* coined as "cinema queerité." This word works so well because it appropriates a former badge of shame and because it suggests that it is not our business or duty to appear acceptable, that there is something inassimilable in nonheterosexuality and only its queerness—its difference—can define it. A similarly differential definition of identity is powerfully articulated in Judith Butler's work, particularly in *Gender Trouble.* Although her final paean to performance has left some unsatisfied with her work's political implications, it is clear that there is something to ponder in the notion that identity (and sex/gender identity in particular) is performative rather than substantive, especially if we remember that a strong sense of discipline would inform any theory of performance, making instantiations or performances of sexuality (queer or straight) more than self-expression.

My point here is not to defend *The Silence of the Lambs.* Its homophobia is apparent *if* by that we mean that it constructs the category of homosexuality within the Symbolic as one marked by pathological lack. In the terms offered us by feminist film theory, we have no feminine object at the center of this spectacle, since Jodie Foster's on-screen presence secures identification rather than specularity, and since the moments of castration are Bill's—when he puts a ring through his tit; when he dances with his cock pulled back between his legs. We have here a spectacle that equates the homosexual with a desire to be a woman and "woman" with castration, and all of that adds up to a pretty oppressive vision of male homosexuality. But how could we expect a narrative about coming of age as an FBI agent to offer anything else? To note this film's homophobia is only to say that it was produced in America. The point in all parables of the law (and this film is nothing if not parabolic of the law of the father) is that no one is free of the implications of any one else's desire or behavior *except* as the mechanisms of identification with the law allow one to fantasize and occupy a social niche securely on this side of transgression. The truly radical response to Demme's film, then, would not be to proclaim its unfairness and misrecognition of homosexual desire (only offered to us through highly coded moments anyway), but rather to suggest that all sexuality is caught within intricate networks of desire and violence, that desire—if never consciously a desire to dismember—always nevertheless dismembers.

Juridically we are subjects marked by our relation to a state that defines us through the criminalization of our sexual behavior—that is one way in which the gay and lesbian struggle is historically different from the struggle of other "minorities." Until those definitions are no longer in force, we cannot forgo the difficult work of identity politics, and that has to include our critique of images from Hollywood and other unenlightened sources. But identity politics as a discourse about juridical subjects keeps us in a definition of power and the political that is monarchical in its origin, keeping us still within what Foucault identifies as "the repressive hypothesis," the notion that power holds in check certain beings—or certain cultural forces like sexuality. In *The History of Sexuality,* Foucault writes that "we must at the same time conceive of sex without the law, and power without the king" (91). The twofold emphasis here is quite important: just as we must think of sexuality without some oppressive law of the father, we must also think it without our own counterlaw. There simply is not some proper, true, pure, or real sexuality waiting to appear once we remove the obstacles of social oppression. Perhaps more crucial to us is Foucault's suggestion that we cannot think power only through "the system of Law-and-Sovereign which has captivated political thought for such a long time" (97). Rather, he writes,

> we need to go one step further, do without the persona of the Prince, and decipher power mechanisms on the basis of a strategy that is immanent in force relationships. . . . In short, it is a question of orienting ourselves to a conception of power which replaces the privilege of law with the viewpoint of the objective, the privilege of prohibition with the viewpoint of tactical efficacy, the privilege of sovereignty with the analysis of a multiple and mobile field of force relations, wherein far-reaching, but never completely stable, effects of domination are produced. (97, 102)

We could think of Foucault's paradigm for the political as postmodern: replacing such stable or foundational discursive politics as Marxism and liberalism (neither of which has been able to formulate a forceful theory of sexuality capable of challenging the privilege of patriarchal masculinity, since the sovereign and his law remain the final referent of all discourse and all bodies in both of these systems) with a reading of power as generalized and diffuse, as immanent in all social relations and therefore variable and reversible. What interests me here is not just the antifoundationalism that drives Foucault's critique of traditional notions of political power but also that his theory deploys itself in terms wholly in accord with contemporary discourses of desire. Power becomes multiple, dispersed, labile, moving across bodies and points of orientation or recognition, marking a struggle between law and aim; this could be Jacques Lacan on desire, but it is Foucault: "a multiple and mobile field of . . . relations, wherein far-reaching, but never completely stable, effects . . . are produced" (102). Foucault challenges us to move out of a stable, dyadic, and ultimately Imaginary understanding of power (including Louis Althusser's reading of ideology and the mirror stage), one that assures subjectivity through the overdetermined presence of a sovereign, transcendent Subject, *and into* a Symbolic universe of discourse where power flows through relations and infuses discourse, knowledge, and subjectivity along channels that are under constant negotiation and renegotiation. Part of what I would like to do here is move beyond an Althusserian notion of the subject and her relation to culture, for as Pierre Bourdieu reminds us, social reality is not simply the reproduction of structures housed in the subject:

> Action is not the mere carrying out of a rule, or obedience to a rule. Social agents, in archaic societies as well as in ours, are not automata regulated like clocks, in accordance with laws they do not understand. In the most complex games, matrimonial exchange for instance, or ritual practices, they put into action the incorporated principles of a generative habitus. . . . This 'feel for the game', as we call it, is what enables an infinite number of 'moves' to be made, adapted to the infinite number of possible situations which no rule, however complex, can foresee. (9)

Thus, identity politics fetishizes not only identity, but also politics to the extent that it imagines social agency as a compulsion within the subject to implicitly obey and act out the power structures that define it *and* to the extent that it essentializes power as the content rather than the generative effect of social relations. What Foucault offers, then, is not just the notion that power is erotic or that sex is ideological (Freud had done that much), but a way of reading power that is fully congruent with our theory of the erotic. His work forces us to consider whether or not homosexual subjectivity—once understood as a self-evidently erotic category—has become part of a taxonomy whose self-evidence is political rather than erotic; and, if any identity politics is bound by the conventions of law rather than desire, then we need to ask whether we have produced in gay and lesbian identity politics a model for thinking about desire that cannot allow desire to operate within it, that cannot (finally) allow for desire. We have to take seriously the possibility that perhaps it has been transgression against sanctioned legal and social identity that has constituted the erotic and seductive appeal of homosexual behavior for many, and that in mapping out new criteria for identification as homosexual, one erases the erotic edge that supposedly is the content of this new subjectivity. In other words, we must face the possibility that the repressed of our canonical moment is erotic pleasure itself (and this is reported as well by older friends who have attended recent Gay Pride activities in New York City only to find that the erotic carnival they participated in in the 1970s—and I mean carnival in the European, Bakhtinian sense—has become a political carnival without the explosive edge of erotic abandon it once allowed).

The final issue I would like to leave you with is the question of agency and how we will think it in the days ahead. Not just through the defunct categories of essential or constructed subjects, not just as automata under a discursive grid more or less hostile to same-sex adventure, but a far more difficult task: to explain our negotiation of the cultural space as a site always still unforeclosed by law; to read in our cognition of ourselves not just the recognition and misrecognition of ourselves and others, but to continue to ask ourselves what—and not just who—queer studies is for. All our profit lies in that asking.

Speaking with the Dead

David Román

What AIDS shows us is the limits of tolerance, that it's not enough to be toler-ated, because when the shit hits the fan you find out how much tolerance is worth. Nothing.—Tony Kushner, *Angels in America*

I feel that my speaking is also disrespectful because it flies in the face of the absoluteness of Tom's death and all the other deaths, as if in the face of that my words could give a sense of closure, of significance, of comfort. In fact, another AIDS death signifies nothing and there isn't or shouldn't be any comfort. So I've made a vow that this is the last memorial at which I will speak.—Robert Rafsky, at fellow AIDS activist Tom Cunningham's memorial

I want to begin by commenting briefly on the epigraphs I have selected to begin my response to Thomas Yingling's "Fetishism, Identity, Poli-tics." Both epigraphs are public performances—one in the theater, the other at an AIDS memorial service—that call attention to the discursive challenges surrounding our relationship to the social phenomenon we call AIDS. In the first, from Tony Kushner's *Angels in America,* Louis (a Jewish gay male who reads Walter Benjamin in bed) speaks to Belize (a black gay man who is a registered nurse and former drag queen). Louis is angry; his lover, Prior, has recently been diagnosed with AIDS. Louis cannot handle Prior's illnesses, but rather than dealing with that directly, he chooses to hold Belize captive in a long exegesis on the problems facing America; his complaint begins with this discussion of the limits of tolerance and his quote on AIDS. As the play continues, it becomes clear that Louis, while insightful, is a talkaholic; Belize tells him so. Louis's main response to AIDS is excessive speech.

The second quote, from Tom Cunningham's memorial service, is spoken by the nationally recognized AIDS activist Robert Rafsky, who died of complications due to AIDS a few weeks later. Rafsky, too, invests in speech. In the memorial to Rafsky published in the *Village Voice,* he is cited as having been one of ACT UP/New York's "most eloquent, and fearless voices" ("Age of AIDS"). Unlike Louis, Rafsky has demonstrated how speech and silence must continually be negotiated in response to AIDS.[1] As his final tribute to Tom Cunningham, Rafsky offers him, and all the others lost to AIDS, his silence. His speaking with the dead is a public performance—indeed, an articulation—of his silence.

I think my responses to AIDS are more often than not caught somewhere between paralysis and agency, between Louis and Rafsky. Beginning about 1980, I started spending time in the theater, and about 1985 I began volunteering for various community AIDS organizations. Both experiences inform how I think and speak, and from both—I don't always separate them so distinctly—I have learned about the function of performativity—that is, of enacting and signifying tactical positions—and about my need for the communal, what Stephen Greenblatt calls, a "felt community" (5). In other words, I too want to speak with the dead. I also want to offer some type of tribute to Thomas Yingling. But I'm not sure how to do either without having my response be, in Rafsky's words and context, "disrespectful." Still, this essay is an attempt to respond to Yingling's ideas, writings, and contributions to lesbian and gay studies, AIDS studies, and American studies. Since it exists in publication, it is also a type of public performance, a performative ritual offered with respect and in recognition of the power of some of those voices now silenced by AIDS but who, despite AIDS, continue to speak to me.

For well over two decades, scholars in all fields—and many with no institutional affiliation (read employment)—have set the groundwork and often the theoretical foundations for the current outpouring of research in lesbian and gay studies. The historian John D'Emilio, among others, has written extensively on these early years of lesbian and gay studies, documenting the various contributions of community-based scholars and their efforts to break down what he sees as the "class-based distinction between intellectual activity and the rest of life" (167).[2] D'Emilio cites a number of interventions—in academic journals, campus life, research institutions, and professional organizations—that have catalyzed the community-based movement of lesbian and gay studies since the 1970s. D'Emilio's history of lesbian and gay studies in the United States forcefully demonstrates that the origins of lesbian and gay studies are unequivocally linked with the post-Stonewall lesbian and gay liberation movement.

Like D'Emilio, Yingling, in "Fetishism, Identity, Politics," writes about this parallel growth of the lesbian and gay movement in and out of American universities and raises serious concerns about the (re)emergence of lesbian and gay studies in the late 1980s. Specifically, Yingling asks us to consider how we might "more critically read the disciplinary or canonical moment of lesbian and gay studies." I suggest we begin to respond to this question by stepping back and speculating on the existence of a "canonical moment" in the first place. I think if we are to understand the current state of gay and lesbian studies, it makes sense to consider the current localized instances of "canonicity" and their relation to the continuing fight for lesbian and gay rights. We need, in short, to account for the locations of lesbian and gay studies: In what departments, institutions, and communities are lesbian and gay studies emerging? If its main harbor is in departments of English or the humanities, what are the limits of this canonical movement?[3] Who and what speaks for lesbian and gay studies in this its most recent manifestation? In what ways do lesbian and gay studies correspond to the national movement for lesbian and gay rights?[4] Undoubtedly, in the 1990s there is more interest in, and tolerance of, the growing industry around lesbian and gay scholarship than twenty years ago, but, as various lesbian and gay scholars and theorists have recently argued, the moment seems anything but canonical.

Lesbians, as usual, run the risk—if not the reality—of being left out of the current wave of interest. Yingling points to this quite clearly when he states that "lesbian and gay studies slips all too easily and all too often into simply 'gay studies,' yet never into 'lesbian studies'" (111; this volume).[5] Julie Abraham goes one step further when she claims that this slippage is a nearly irreparable dilemma intrinsic to the discipline as it was formulated in the 1980s: "A gay/lesbian studies identified with the subject of sexuality will inevitably favor gay subjects, even when the emphasis is on the perverse and the queer, because the culture's discussion of sexual dissidence has been so consistently a discussion of the homosexual male" (21). She joins Elizabeth Grosz who, in "Bodies and Pleasures in Queer Theory," also questions why lesbianism has been "so decidedly ignored" (226).

If we are left to wonder, as Yingling insists we must, what is being repressed in the canonical moment of lesbian and gay studies, it may well be lesbians or, as Sue-Ellen Case explains, certain kinds of lesbians. Case argues that whatever new lesbian visibility there is in the 1990s is premised on the "lesbian with phallus-as-fetish," the lesbian with a dildo who is "born out of the rib of gay male subcultural images" (39). This lesbian, according to Case, emerges out of the cultural logic of phallic (re)production. Such a normalizing logic allows for the location of the newfound lesbian visibility in a limited representational economy that can only reabsorb her within the specific agendas of its ideological authority. Case explains the illusion of power created by this process: "While the dyke believes she is finally appearing, she is actually disappearing into the market" (45). Thus, she concludes, "when the dyke enters the class(room), she is on the stage of dominant practices" (45), a stage with little room for, or tolerance of, the order of lesbian politics.

In an essay that shares some of these concerns but focuses primarily on the need to address issues of race and ethnicity in lesbian and gay studies, Yvonne Yarbro-Bejarano explains how lesbians of color—both in and out of the classroom—stand outside of this representational and critical commodification process, unimagined at worst or visualized only within the normative racialized discourses of white fetishistic erotics at best. Like Abraham and Case, Yarbro-Bejarano raises serious and as yet unanswered concerns regarding the idea of a "canonical moment" in lesbian and gay studies. Yarbro-Bejarano calls for a lesbian and gay studies that includes more than "just white, middle-class lesbians and gays" (126). By offering a means for imagining such a field (see also Román), she challenges us to recognize and "emphasize the contribution of lesbians of color to this theoretical project of categorical expansion, in part because some white feminists have appropriated that contribution, and also because lesbians of color have provided a significant piece of the theoretical groundwork that could and should serve as the foundation of lesbian and gay studies" (130). Yarbro-Bejarano, for example, cites the work of a number of Chicana lesbians—Cherríe Moraga, Gloria Anzaldúa, Chela Sandoval—who provide a new paradigm for understanding marginality and oppression by theorizing their "multiple and shifting identities and identifications, consciousness, and political agency" (133). Yarbro-Bejarano's project begins to enact the more critical readings of lesbian and gay studies suggested in Yingling's essay, demonstrating, along with Abraham, Case, and Grosz, the type of work lesbian and gay scholars have yet to do.

More to the point, these diverse lesbian theorists call into question the by now commonplace assumption that lesbian and gay studies has found its niche in academic institutions. The fact that there is *already* in place a location from which to challenge the critical authority emerging within (as) lesbian and gay studies in no way undermines the significance of their concerns. To speak about lesbian and gay studies, especially within academic forums such as this one, more often than not presupposes an unproblematic positionality for the field. The act of speaking, seemingly validated with publication, suggests the illusion of an arrival at once welcome and stable—despite the subjectivity and concerns of the speaker—simply on the basis that something has been said, even if this something is actually a critique of the very process that allows its articulation in the first place. Therefore, lesbian voices such as these—the malcontents at the annual cashbar—may be expected, perhaps even tolerated, but not without some price for both speaker and listener. "Can we talk?" asks Marlon Riggs, "but of course we can, queer diva darling, if you abide by the rules of dominant discourse, which means in short, you must ultimately sing somebody else's tune to be heard" (101). The apprehensions voiced by white lesbian theorists and lesbian and gay theorists of color—each with distinct relationships to the university—suggest both the limits of the "canonical" and the complexity of effects associated with the practice of lesbian and gay studies.

This is especially true if we consider the position of lesbian and gay studies for students. I imagine that Riggs's comments hold particular resonance for queer graduate students of all genders and colors who must practice what he calls "verbal drag schtick," the haunting self-conscious activity of second guessing and performing critical authorities in order to legitimate one's own speaking position: "But does she comprehend discursive intertextual analysis, can she engage in postfeminist, neo-Marxist, postmodern deconstructionist critique? Does she understand the difference between text, subtext, and metatext?" (Riggs 103).

Despite what Michael Warner describes as the "boom point" ("From Queer" 19) in the field, out lesbian and gay scholars negotiating graduate exam reading lists, dissertation committees, research grants, reappointment and tenure rulings are continually vulnerable to the muscle of individual and institutional homophobia prevalent throughout the academy. A career based in lesbian and gay studies still holds no guarantees. A simple perusal of recent Modern Language Association's (MLA) job lists will counter any notions of canonicity. Are two or three job-listings a year advertising for an *interest* in lesbian and gay studies enough to constitute a significant breakthrough? I remember how quickly my enthusiasm for these few positions dissipated when I noticed how many other institutions were not searching for their "queer theorist." D'Emilio claims that with the new market interest in lesbian and gay scholarship, "a young lesbian and gay scholar may have difficulty finding a job, but she or he is increasingly likely to have a dissertation published" (168). True, perhaps, but notice too the scholar's "difficulty finding a job." Only here does publication without employment threaten the possibility of actually landing a teaching position.[6]

Even those who have established the critical vocabularies of the profession and have been rewarded with tenure are not exempt from constant surveillance and attack. The public gay-baiting of Professor David Halperin (an internationally respected scholar and pioneer in the field) in response to slanderous and unsubstantiated accusations against him by a disgruntled colleague at MIT demonstrates the vulnerability we all face in practicing and promoting lesbian and gay studies on our campuses.[7] Capitalizing on that campaign of vilification, Roger Kimball bashed Halperin in the *Wall Street Journal* while covering the 1992 MLA conference: "A great deal that Prof. Halperin had to say about sex that afternoon cannot be printed in a family newspaper. But it is worth reminding ourselves that his students at MIT regularly receive his unedited reflections on this and other subjects in his classes. Tuition at MIT is $18,000 a year. I wonder if the parents of MIT students think they are getting value for their money." While many would want to dismiss such a personal attack as typical of a certain extremist position in the popular press, Kimball's comments suggest the kinds of attitudes gay and lesbian scholars continually confront.[8]

The fundamental point I want to make is that the current interest in, and controversies around, lesbian and gay studies cannot be understood in isolation from other discursive practices addressing lesbians, gays, and queers. Just as the emergence of a critical practice identified as "lesbian and gay studies" and the theoretical arsenal now readily understood as "queer theory" needs to be seen in conjunction with other political and social movements in gay and lesbian life in the 1990s, as D'Emilio suggests, so must the attacks against gay and lesbian scholars and scholarship be viewed as yet one more salient display of bias and hatred informing the national debates on lesbian and gay civil rights.

D'Emilio explains the importance of understanding the dynamics of the university as a social space informed by and participating in the ideological practices of its day. He writes: "One of the signal achievements of the campus turmoil of the 1960s was the recognition that universities are not ivory towers where individuals engage in the disinterested, dispassionate, and detached pursuit of knowledge and truth. Rather, universities are intimately connected to the society of which they are a part. They are capable of producing change, to be sure, but they also reflect, and reproduce, the dominant values, beliefs, habits, and inequalities of their society" (162).

The current status of lesbians and gays in the United States remains under serious debate. The "boom" in queer theory, and in lesbian and gay studies in general, is in many ways symptomatic of these debates, as Grosz explains in "Bodies and Pleasures in Queer Theory." To identify the moment in gay and lesbian studies as "canonical" invents a legitimating space not always available for many of the lesbian and gay scholars I have cited. It presupposes secured political positions for gays and lesbians inside and outside of the university and imagines commodity fetishism and the rhetoric of tolerance as viable sites for lesbian and gay agency. The task at hand is to critically locate sites of agency in order to challenge the commodification and depoliticization of lesbian and gay studies within institutional movements based on tolerance or market trends.

While Yingling sees the late 1980s as the canonical moment in lesbian and gay studies and introduces this theme by citing the cultural anthropologist and theorist James Clifford, I view the late 1980s and early 1990s as a liminal movement in lesbian and gay studies. I want to cite a different anthropologist, Victor Turner, to make my point. Turner explains that "the attributes of liminality are necessarily ambiguous, since the condition and the persons elude or slip through the networks of classifications that normally locate states and positions in cultural space" (95). Liminality suggests the neither here nor there; it insists on the *process* of social initiation, the ways in which cultures enact legitimacy and authority and acculturate subjects into the social fabric of its reigning ideology. Turner, of course, builds upon the ideas of Arnold Van Gennep, who introduces the concept of the liminal to theorize social "rites of passage." For both Van Gennep and Turner, the liminal is the transitional moment between

> [an] earlier fixed state in the social structure, from a set of cultural conditions (a "state"), or from both. During the intervening "liminal" period, the characteristics of the ritual subject (the "passenger") are ambiguous; he passes through a cultural realm that has few or none of the attributes of the past or coming state. In the third phrase (reaggregation or reincorporation), the passage is consummated. The ritual subject, individual or corporate, is in a relatively stable state once more and, by virtue of this, has rights and obligations vis-à-vis others of a clearly defined and "structural" type; he is expected to behave in accordance with certain customary norms and ethical standards binding on incumbents of social position in a system of such positions. (Turner 94–95)

I invoke the less fashionable ideas of Van Gennep and Turner because it may be precisely within this border space of the liminal that pleasure itself can be recuperated for lesbian and gay studies—recuperated, that is, if we agree with Yingling that erotic pleasure has been repressed in lesbian and gay studies. Yingling worries that "we must face the possibility that the repressed of our canonical moment is erotic pleasure itself" (117; this volume) and cites both the institutionalization of lesbian and gay studies and the political investment in identity politics as complicit in this process. His suggestion that we more critically examine the "canonical moment" must involve then a process of locating the erotic and pleasurable in lesbian and gay studies.

Some have found pleasure in the dynamics of the classroom. For Joseph Litvak, for example, pleasure may be recuperated through the teaching of lesbian and gay studies.[9] Working within the Foucauldian model that frames Yingling's essay, Litvak reminds us that the same system that produces discipline must also produce " 'perversions,' if only to encrypt them in each and every good middle-class subject as so many stages (suggestive term) through which he or she must pass" (10). Litvak suggests that it is precisely at this moment of encrypting that lesbian and gay studies can intervene: teaching gay studies "seems, that is, to offer a way of prying open the crypts that have already been sealed, of keeping others from forming too quickly, of bringing out, or educing, or even educating loves, pleasures, and desires that education otherwise serves to put away" (11). Litvak's goal for lesbian and gay studies is to recognize the ideological processes that produce surveillance and transgression, including the university and the classroom, and to identify and extend the moments—what I would call liminal moments—when these positions are negotiated.[10]

If the liminal performs the not yet disciplined, the almost disciplined, the about to be disciplined, it makes sense for us to exploit it. Rather than aiming toward the canonical, it may be worthwhile to protract the liminal moment of lesbian and gay studies. Judith Butler has taught us that it is often politically efficacious for us *as* lesbians and gays to "proliferate and intensify the crisis of identity politics" ("Force of Fantasy" 121), to allow for and revel in the anxieties or pleasures produced by the "uncontrollability" of the categorical terms established by regulatory disciplines and institutions. I find Butler's response to the crisis of identity politics remarkably useful in thinking through the current status of lesbian and gay studies. If lesbian and gay studies is in the liminal phase—a process that gestures toward, and at times even aspires to, the canonical—and if the liminal is defined inherently as uncategorical, then the possibilities of our scholarship and pedagogy and their effects are endless. It is precisely in the intensification of the liminal where the proliferation of multiple subjectivities, multiple *kinds* of lesbian and gay studies, and multiple pleasures become available to us. The liminal phase always enacts the move toward canonicity: it produces the illusion of assimilation while still holding license to remain temporarily outside of disciplinary control, even as it presupposes a narrative that will conclude in the initiation of customary norms.

From this perspective, the current crisis in lesbian and gay studies seems less about the anxiety of who and what queer studies is for or about. Rather it seems to me that the crisis is located in the institutional demands that insist upon responses to such questions: institutional demands that arrive in the form of justifications for new programs, courses, and hires from not always sympathetic deans, chairs, and colleagues. These demands are further exacerbated by the local governing bodies of higher education, especially for publicly funded state schools and institutions with religious affiliations. Lesbians and gays know only too well that there are few, if any, discursive ways out of inquiries pertaining to sexuality that are not already predetermined and contained within dominant discourse or, in Yingling's words, "unforeclosed by law" (117; this volume). How can we possibly answer these questions—who and what queer studies is for and about—without falling into either the trap of defensive rhetoric or the universalizing, but well-intended, impulse of bourgeois liberalism?

It is not possible to escape these questions: Who is queer studies for? What is queer studies for? Yingling concludes his essay by challenging us with his proposal that "all our profit lies in that asking." The multiple, shifting identities that each of us may bring at any time to our classrooms, institutions, and communities, with students, peers, and colleagues—whether queer or straight and with differing degrees of homophobia and homoignorance—suggest that these questions will always be asked and answered differently depending upon the local circumstances and specific dynamics of the exchange. This is not to say that these questions are trivial. I agree with Yingling that it is to our profit that we consider the purposes of our practices. But these questions can only be addressed locally and always in consideration of the materiality of who can speak. Our responses will never be choral and will differ according to our own specific circumstances and subject positions.

Yet, what are the limits of celebrating the liminal if as lesbians and gays we continue to aspire to a type of acculturation, with all the customary norms—domestic partnership, antidiscrimination, and other civil rights—available and intact? I think Yingling offers us a way to conceptualize a response that allows for both the radical capacities of the liminal and the securing comforts of the canonical when he writes that "our discourse and our being are not organic appearances but arise at the nexus of other forms of knowledge, power, and pleasure, and our analysis of homosexuality or homophobia needs always to inquire into this structural density" (111; this volume). Lesbian and gay studies, to prove successful in the long run, must continue to recognize and explore what Yingling refers to and what Yarbro-Bejarano explicates more fully: that our identities and our desires, while based historically in marginalization and oppression, are dynamic processes that escape the construction of a "distinct culture."

While Yingling and Yarbro-Bejarano, among others, provide the theoretical framework for lesbian and gay studies, it is important to note that AIDS activists have provided a menu of available tactics that may enable social change for gays and lesbians inside and outside of the university. While AIDS, according to Kushner, has shown us the limits of tolerance, AIDS activists have demonstrated the efficacy of local interventions against the systemic processes that discriminate against people with AIDS and contribute to the growing epidemic (see Crimp, *AIDS*). Such "local resistances" contest the systems of power that construct and, in the process, control marginal identities. As Cindy Patton explains:

> The idea of local resistances, taken seriously and in specific contexts, means that coalition, especially geographically understood, is not a coherent idea. What the emergence of ACT UP through the silence = death symbols suggests is that sparks are given off through attempts to "unleash" power within the power/discourse gap. Resistance in other locales may be ignited by these sparks, but must spring from an analysis of the local situation, finding leverage points within the narrow space offered differently by different localities. (163)

Patton's ideas on the local claim highlight the necessity to intervene on multiple fronts differently—perhaps even in contradiction or, using her term, "incoherent[ly]"—*and* to recognize that there are always multiple, distinct sites of contestation. She recommends that activists focus on tactics and locality and then strategize accordingly. This is good advice and an excellent program for lesbian and gay studies if we are to make a dent in the always different institutional biases leveled against us. There is no reason, as D'Emilio has argued consistently, for scholars to view the university as any more accommodating than any other social institution or discipline. For those who work in lesbian and gay studies, the task remains both to exploit and maintain the liminal phase of lesbian and gay studies and to work directly in our local environments to systematically challenge and contest institutional regimes that, at best, tolerate our presence and scholarship.[11] Such a simultaneous endeavor, while employing particular tactics of resistance for different localities, only demonstrates the need to engage the multiple sites of contestation within the university.

But there is more at stake for lesbian and gay studies at this point than simply replicating and appropriating the tactics of AIDS activists in order to challenge the local instances and dynamics of regulatory violence normalized against queers in the 1990s. We must also keep the focus on AIDS as a priority agenda of lesbian and gay studies, for as Simon Watney explains, "we should not define lesbian and gay studies in a way which marginalizes an epidemic that is undoubtedly the worst single catastrophe in 'our' history, however we theorize 'ourselves'" ("Lesbian and Gay Studies" 72). A thorough and interdisciplinary analysis of AIDS is still needed if we are to understand the often contradictory ways AIDS is both constructed and encountered in different locales and communities, the effective and noneffective counterstrategies in local resistances employed to fight AIDS, and the various power networks (including the university and its production of knowledge) by which their effects are extended. Such work necessitates, as Butler explains in her support of Watney's position, "an important set of dialogues among those who work between the academy and the movement to think about priorities" ("Letter"). These dialogues among people with different and multiple positionalities, subjectivities, and desires will facilitate both our understanding of and response to AIDS, as well as serve as a tribute to the dead, especially to those who helped establish initially the lesbian and gay studies we profess to practice.

I never met Thomas Yingling, although we were scheduled to meet at the MLA in New York in 1992. I had organized a panel, through the Gay and Lesbian Caucus of the MLA, on "AIDS: Politics and Pedagogies in the University," and Yingling was set to deliver the paper abstracted in this volume ("AIDS, Confession, and Theory") on teaching with AIDS. He died some months before the meeting. Our only immediate connection during his life was through our correspondence. I think, although I'm not really sure, that we may have gotten along, but the possibility of a conversation, never mind a friendship, is now foreclosed by AIDS. Or is it? How peculiar is it for me to continue responding to Tom (can I call him Tom?) knowing, of course, all along that he is dead. How, after all, can we speak, indeed argue, with the dead? Because of our overlapping and nearly historical conjunction as gay men in the academy interested in lesbian and gay studies, and despite our significant differences—in rank and status, race and ethnicity, professional interests and training, and most acutely, our relationship to AIDS—I want to claim an affinity with him. I realize, of course, that in the process of identification I run the risk of enacting the very violence of misrecognition he has argued so effectively against. This, for me, is an acceptable and worthwhile risk, for how else can I convey and indulge my romantic impulse for what could have been and my relentless rage for what will never be?

To speak and identify as someone who is not living with AIDS assumes, inevitably and unfortunately, a desire to differentiate from people with AIDS. For a gay man (and one of color) to announce publicly his seronegativity (however tenuous this may be)[12] plays into a dynamic established by the dominant discursive strategies that constructs people with AIDS as other. It perpetuates the very problematic and omnipresent binarism (usually at the expense of people with AIDS) that insistently categorizes people as with AIDS or without.[13] This is not my aim. I am left wondering what means are available to me to speak with the dead—to claim an identification—without enacting the violence of misrecognition. Can there be recognition without violence? Is my mourning only a narcissistic performance of survival? Or, if I am speaking with the dead, who is listening and what is the response? All my profit lies in this asking.

Notes

This essay was written in the spring of 1993. Discussions with Carolyn Dinshaw, Yvonne Yarbro-Bejarano, Robyn Wiegman, and David Norton have helped shape some of these ideas. I would also like to thank Sue-Ellen Case, Yvonne Yarbro-Bejarano, Brad Epps, and Joe Litvak for sharing with me the early drafts of their essays.

1   For me, the most useful discussions of this negotiation are Sedgwick, "White Glasses"; Crimp, "Right On, Girlfriend!"; and Harper.

2   See also Escoffier, who constructs a less dynamic history of the field by insisting on the binarism not only between two, for him, distinct generations of scholars but also between those inside and outside of the academy.

3   See Epps, for example, who discusses this in relation to Spanish traditions, and Easton, who provides a thorough discussion of gay and lesbian studies and art history. This is not to suggest, by any means, that the social sciences and other disciplines have not engaged lesbian and gay issues. It is precisely the question as to how this work is eclipsed by the humanities, and more specifically "English," that I wish to raise.

4   On this point, see the interview with Duberman where he recounts how in Vermont, a conservative politician after reading Duberman's coedited anthology, *Hidden from History: Reclaiming the Lesbian and Gay Past*, helped rally support for the success of the lesbian and gay state civil rights bill.

5   Although Yingling calls attention to the "repression" of the lesbian in *lesbian and* gay studies, his essay simultaneously enacts it by claiming a canonical moment for lesbian and gay studies.

6   Yingling refers to this problem in his earlier essay, "Sexual Preference/ Cultural Reference." He writes: "to be openly gay or lesbian in the academy, to be working on gay and lesbian literature and theory (despite what seems to be something of a revolution in manners), is still to find oneself all too often embattled, belittled, and un(der)employed" (94; this volume).

7   For a detailed discussion of Halperin's situation, see Nussbaum. Unfortunately, Nussbaum, in an otherwise brilliant argument, does not factor in lesbian studies.

8   In a letter to the editor of the *Wall Street Journal* (27 Jan. 1993), Timothy B. Peters, a former student of Halperin's, protested against Kimball's insinuations: "Mr. Kimball makes a leap by assuming that radical scholarship automatically translates into radical and/or bad teaching. . . . To suggest that radical fields of inquiry discredit a scholar's ability to teach (an often altogether different pursuit) makes the criticism personal and meanspirited and, therefore, inappropriate."

Degrees of homophobia are also omnipresent in the publishing world. Richard Mohr, for example, sees this as the central problem he encountered in his attempts to find a university press to publish his recent book *Gay Ideas: Outing and Other Controversies.* The anthology *How Do I Look? Queer Film and Video,* edited by Bad Object-Choices and published by Seattle's Bay Press, could not find a domestic printer. In both cases, presses and printers were concerned primarily with images discussed and reproduced in the texts.

9   Litvak's paper, incidentally, was presented at a 1992 MLA panel sponsored by the Gay and Lesbian Caucus whose call for papers was entitled "Classrooms from Hell." By the time of the meeting, the program was retitled "Mourning, Shaming, Trashing, and Pogroms in and around the Queer Studies Classroom." The other presenters were Michèle Aina Barale, Sean Holland, and Eve Kosofsky Sedgwick.

10 And yet, it needs to be noted, Litvak joins Sue-Ellen Case in pointing out the vexed position of the lesbian or gay teacher in the classroom.

11 Consider for example two completely different and simultaneous occasions for lesbian and gay studies. In 1992, the Center for Lesbian and Gay Studies under the direction of Martin Duberman at the Graduate School of the City University of New York received a $250,000 Rockefeller grant. That same year the Auburn Gay and Lesbian Association (AGLA), a queer student group at Auburn University in Alabama, was denied access to university funds since AGLA supposedly advocated the violation of state sodomy laws. The Alabama state senate unanimously approved this censure.

12   Once again, I cite Sedgwick's "White Glasses" for an excellent discussion of the tenuous nature of speaking subjects and (our) health, in particular as it relates to our positions around HIV and AIDS.

13   See, for instance and for starters, Sullivan, "Gay Life, Gay Death." Moreover, to test positive for human immunodeficiency virus (HIV) is not the same as to be diagnosed with AIDS. In other words, HIV and AIDS are not coterminous and/or interchangeable terms.

Untitled

These scars I carry on my body
are but the latest indication
you on one side of things, me on the other.

It could be a dream
in which I see this,
but we have become too worldly to believe
that dreams are not of this world.

Certainly it is recurrent,
and everyone is in profile,
as on coins. This has a history
I cannot excavate without you. . . .

The Stuttering I

Theory and the Debate over Canon

In 1929, Gertrude Stein had a terrible fight with Bernard Fay over nouns and adjectives. She didn't like them, she said, and he did. She punished him by making his portrait almost entirely of adverbs and prepositions in *How Writing Is Written*. It was no doubt not with our present quandary over canons and canonicity in view that Wallace Stevens in 1942 resolved the problem of choice and all the binary heritage of Western metaphysics by declaiming: "it was not a choice / Between excluding things. It was not a choice / / Between, but of" ("Notes Toward a Supreme Fiction" 403).

But Stevens's resolution speaks to the problem we wish to solve in literary study today: too often we think of the choices of canonicity as terribly urgent, and we tend to structure those as choices "between" and not "of," as choices of either/or rather than and/and. Only so much can be taught, the pragmatic argument runs, and some exclusions must be made. The Stevens choice "to include the things / That in each other are included, the whole, / The complicate, the amassing harmony" (403), cannot be our choice. We haven't the luxury of time necessary to attend "the whole, the complicate, the amassing harmony" except as specialists, especially since the problem of canonicity finds its most naturalized site in the classroom, where such grand schemes of harmony are exactly what we wish to challenge in our students' naive assumptions about literary history. The whole thrust of poststructuralist debate—and we will include the issue of canonicity in that debate for the moment—has been to question the legitimacy of that vision of literary history suggested by Stevens: there is no whole, complicate, or amassing harmony except as certain voices are forced to harmonize, except as others are silenced or ignored.

The debate over canonicity has raged for quite a few years now in literary circles, but I for one am not sure that it is a useful question anymore, that it indeed helps us to do the work that needs to be done in overturning notions of "the amassing harmony." We have not solved the problem of the canon's past exclusivity simply by offering seminars on women poets whose work was written out of former literary histories, for instance; and we can offer anthologies that include—or champion—Afro-American, Commonwealth, Amerasian and Amerindian writers, women, gay men, and lesbians, but the anthology enforces a particular way of reading texts and is still a benign prison for those tokenized in it. In neither of these cases have we eliminated the problem that produced our desire for a canon in the first place. Too often we relegate the debate over canonicity to a problem of literary history and rewrite that history more inclusively, but the question facing us is not really "which poets ought we to teach" (and I take it here that poetry, unlike fiction and drama, exists in America almost exclusively within academic markets that choose to produce and reproduce certain texts and not others)—the question is, rather, "why are we teaching poetry at all?" Is there room, need, or use for poetry in the curriculum? Before we can ask whether some do it better, differently, or more to our liking than others, we need to decide what it—poetry—does.

I will turn to this point later but wish to demonstrate first how debates over canonicity produce conservative ends not congruent with their liberal beginnings when they do not address the more fundamental problem of what poetry can do that other texts cannot. We all know that canons are political, for instance, that they serve "the dominant interests." But what those dominant interests are is not always apparent—or is, I should say, perhaps most to be questioned when they appear most natural and self-evident.

Let us take the issue of gender, the issue that has perhaps had the most telling impact on the question of canon in American literature. The "dominant interest" in the field of gender is the interest of the patriarchy, of course, and I do not for a moment mean to diminish or question how hegemonic and oppressive is the system of institutions and ideological apparatuses that constitute patriarchal control. But the way in which this problem is translated into the issue of canon debate cannot simply be to see the problem as one of representation, of making sure that women receive equal time and pay (in the form of articles, conferences, and appearances on the syllabus). This constitutes part of Marjorie Perloff's critique of Sandra Gilbert and Susan Gubar's *Norton Anthology of Literature By Women*—that too often, its choices seem to be made primarily on the basis of gender and with little consideration given to questions of aesthetics (see Perloff). I am not about to suggest that aesthetics escape ideology or that our thinking about canon should be based in aesthetic concerns: surely, that is exactly what we have been fighting against. But Perloff is persuasive in her critique of Gilbert and Gubar because she introduces us to the work of a poet excluded by them (Lorrine Niedecker) whose work in Objectivist conventions interrogates the position of women in patriarchal structure, but does so in an aesthetic that challenges the reader in a way foreign to many of the more overtly "political" and "feminist" texts included in Gilbert and Gubar's anthology.

Perloff's main point of contention is not that Gilbert and Gubar have overlooked a significant voice (although her essay makes a case for reevaluating Niedecker's lack of reputation); rather, her essay asks that feminist criticism address the problem of subjectivity in a more poststructuralist manner than it often currently does in constructing its own, "alternative" canon. Cora Kaplan's argument in "Pandora's Box" is more pointed:

> as I see it, the present danger is not that feminist criticism will enter an unequal dependent alliance with any of the varieties of male-centered criticism. It does not need to, for it has produced an all too persuasive autonomous analysis which is in many ways radical in its discussion of gender, but implicitly conservative in its assumptions about social hierarchy and female subjectivity.... Humanist feminist criticism does not object to the idea of an immanent, transcendent subject but only to the exclusion of women from these definitions which it takes as an accurate account of subjectivity rather than as a historically constructed ideology.

> The repair and reconstitution of female subjectivity through a
> rereading of literature becomes, therefore, a major part, often un-
> acknowledged, of its critical project. (147, 149)

What Kaplan identifies here is exactly the point: our debate over canonicity often is so complicit with humanist assumptions about literary
texts, their place and value in culture, that it is little more than a
rearrangement of issues that accord completely with the social fabric
of American postcapitalism (I see this most clearly on a personal and
professional level in the astonishing recent explosion of publishing for
a gay market—almost all of which understands the political agenda of
homosexuality from a liberal, democratic point of view, and much of
which is completely bourgeois in its values). The debate needs to shift,
at this point, from the problem of which texts are read to the question
of how any text is produced and reproduced within and against a
number of ideological constructions and constraints.

Wendy Martin's *American Triptych* is exemplary of the desire to
restructure our understanding of American poetic history according to
the issues of gender, but it certainly becomes at points an example of
Kaplan's complaint, accepting the notion of the immanent, transcendent subject as "an accurate account of subjectivity rather than as a
historically constructed ideology." Martin's work compares the constraints historically faced by women writers to the freedom men have
had, using (at one point) Adrienne Rich and Allen Ginsberg as examples. In this particular comparison, men's writing is characterized as
egocentric and women's as "concerned with internal process and relationship" (199), and her examples do indeed point to these qualities in
the texts of Ginsberg and Rich. Martin sees Ginsberg as "the death
knell of the male counterculture," moving eccentrically around the
globe in his phallocratic freedom, while Rich, the martyr, is "fran-
tically writing poetry between household chores or in the middle of
the night after comforting a restless child" (198). The problem here is
not just the oversimplification of her comparison (I oversimplify her
text to make my point), nor even that Martin should perhaps have
examined Ginsberg's compromised phallocentrism, his "queer" position in the patriarchy (this is his term).

The real problem is that Martin as critic has become transparent to
the egos her analysis encounters. She takes her position as reader by
identifying with "Ginsberg" and "Rich," and does not see "them" as
textual effects but as egos with fulfilled or stifled potentials for tran-

scendent self-expression. I realize that we have here the specter of a man speaking woman's most useful desire for her, and I regret that I cast myself in this position; as a male teacher with feminist concerns, I am aware of the dangers in this position. But I use Martin as an example here not because I wish to cast aspersions on the feminist project but to point toward one of the avenues that project (and the related projects of gay/lesbian and Afro-American studies) can no longer afford to take (and, indeed, it seems less and less to be taking this approach). I wish to raise the question that is bracketed in discussions ending with a call for "equal time" according to race, gender, class, or ethnicity: that is, what do we consider the use and value of poetry to be, and why should it be part of a curriculum at all?

Do we believe, for instance, that studying poetry can make one a better human being, a better woman, a better citizen, a more liberal or enlightened American? To answer "yes" to any of these is to see poetry as the site of the production of a surplus value that accrues to the individual who consumes it. It is still to buy into the myth of literature as ennobling. But why is reading a poem more ennobling than studying automobile designs of the 1950s? What is the value of reading Sylvia Plath if one does not understand the crisis of legitimation that is so ingrained in her text? Can her poems teach our students to navigate the treacherous shoals of postindustrial capitalism and the narrow straits of postheterosexuality? Before we can decide what canon is acceptable (and Plath is part of mine because she so systematically overturns our expectations of centered subjectivity), we must decide "acceptable for what?" (I take it here that to say we will not have a canon is impossible; choices are made according to interested positions, and we are each covalent with at least one interested position. We each have a canon.) What is it we are trying to teach when we teach poetry? Is it coverage—a comprehensive understanding of twentieth-century poetry? Why? Is it an in-depth study of some minds we find of value (leading to seminars on Frank O'Hara, Elizabeth Bishop, or Gwendolyn Brooks)? Why? Is it politics or gender we consider important? (Might Robert Lowell enter here?) Or is it class? (Might Robert Lowell enter here?) Or are we trying still to teach something captured in the word "poetics," an appreciation of form and structure, the empty center from which all illusion is called forth? (Might Robert Lowell figure here?)

I, for one, can find value in any or all of the above projects for study, but I can no longer take for granted that such projects are self-evidently meaningful or important, and I refuse to grant that they are revisionist of the canon simply because they include sections on feminism or place Elizabeth Bishop in equal relation to Wallace Stevens. Our purpose in reforming the canon of modernist poetry oughtn't to be simply getting rid of T. S. Eliot or showing up his misogyny. We cannot solve the problem of Eliot simply by also reading H.D. Our critique needs to be of ideology and the needs it inscribes in us as readers, scholars, and teachers even when our politics are noble and liberationist. Perhaps the thing to say about Eliot at this time, for instance, does not primarily concern gender (although certainly his text exhibits a radical misogyny that cannot be ignored) but focuses on class—on the dynamic of an "allusive" tradition that is a literary enactment of the social desire for inheritance. Eliot (and Ezra Pound with him) speak an aristocratic tongue wherein Greek and Latin are inherited as the signs of textual class just as property, houses, manners, and style are inherited as signs of economic and social class. It seems that we do not so much need to rid the canon of Eliot and Pound as we need to use them to say something about the canon's ideological interests.

Certainly a crucial aspect of those interests concerns gender. That men have been more generally inheritors of all signs of culture and plenty would have to be addressed in this, as well as the fact that Eliot misrecognizes the problem of the "modern" as the problem of private sexual relations. But part of what is at stake in reforming our reading practices of Eliot, Pound, or any other male modernist must be related to class, and to the interconnections between class and gender—including our critical misrecognition of the one for the other. Frank Lentricchia's essay on Wallace Stevens in *Critical Inquiry,* "Patriarchy Against Itself," makes a case for the intertextuality of inheritance, economic self-reliance, literary authority, and gender in American modernism, and while one can critique the essay (as Gilbert and Gubar rightly do in "The Man on the Dump") for its "testerical" attack on essentialist feminism or for its acceptance of Oedipus, an acceptance that inevitably naturalizes heterosexual deployments of desire, one must still recognize that Lentricchia's text begins to ask a new question about Stevens. (Ann Kibbey's work in earlier American literature takes a similar, more explicitly "feminist" approach, and Cora Kaplan is exemplary in this.) The books and essays of these critics could not be written today if it were not for the work of liberal feminists who in the dozen years since Kate Millett's *Sexual Politics* have made gender a canonical issue. But such work goes beyond the limitations of humanist feminism and places gender as one function within a more complex understanding of the social fields of discourse and control.

My point here is that "fixing" the canon will not do—not just because it will still be "fixed" (i.e., immobile and hegemonic)—but more importantly because the canon is not the problem. The real problem we face, as teachers, writers, and scholars interested in poetry is that we can no longer teach "poetry." Let us think, for instance, of a course in modern and postmodern American poetry that centers on the problem of the object; and let us think of this as the enlightened project of a postformalist, post-"authorial" teacher. Certainly, we would find Pound at the core of such a course; we would read Fenellosa and Eliot and look at the theory of the image and of the objective correlative. We might use Williams, and those who wanted to address gender would ask why the objects in those other texts were always so insistently female and/ or feminized. We could bring in Marianne Moore's work and perhaps Elizabeth Bishop's mapping, Sylvia Plath's horrific rooms full of threat, or Lorrine Niedecker's long canonical silence (if they'd heard of her through Marjorie Perloff). The course could also include Objectivists—Denise Levertov, Robert Creeley—and could look at Afro-American traditions for depicting objects of desire (Langston Hughes's "Trumpet Player," for instance). It might even return at some point to the good old Canon Aspirin's author, Wallace Stevens. But what would such a course have accomplished? As I have described it here, it would have made the desire to possess, describe, and/or essentialize objects the natural center of consciousness, shared equally if differently (and in such cases difference is used only to establish deeper similarities) among all people. It would place the poet still at the center of a linguistic system he or she controls, and the inevitable point about the resistance of things to language would have made poetry's existence that much more mysterious, would have made the poem itself as object a very special case.

How different this same course would feel if it began *not* with the object as given (even when questioned as to gender) but with the object as a question, with Roland Barthes's *Mythologies* and the analysis of objects as ideological markers, with the altogether astonishing analyses of Baudrillard into the way objects reify ideological positions, with Lacan's "*objet petit a*" or Julia Kristeva's psycho-semiotics. Such a course would no longer be "English 393" or "Contemporary American Poetry." It would have become something concerned with the theory of poetry *as language* and with the inscription of objects both in and as texts. It would include Gertrude Stein's "Tender Buttons" and Hart Crane's "Possessions." It would analyze the construction of desiring subjects and their objects of desire according to gender expectations; it might even employ films. This is the course we need, I would argue, one that moves beyond the question of canon (because canon is always bound by genre, nation, gender, a naive relationality to history; even revisionist canons reify their texts as natural expressions of human interest) into the question of representation itself. Such a course would encounter the question of textuality, subjectivity, and semiotics; it would investigate difference (including sexual difference) as the constitutive stuff of writing.

Oh, you say, that sounds like a course on theory and not a course on poetry. But this is exactly my point. The debate over whether or not theory deserves a central place in our curriculum, and what its impact on the liberal art of literary study would be, is still a question that is bracketed and glossed over in our work when we allow debates over canonicity to absorb our attention without thinking of them within the problematic of discursive representation. Theory begins the project that grants the problem of canonicity meaning and yet is forced to remain conveniently beyond its horizon. But it is precisely the value of poetry for our teaching at this time that it leads directly into a confrontation with the subject as an ideological effect of theories of language. In *Mythologies,* Roland Barthes writes:

> Contemporary poetry . . . tries to transform the sign back into meaning: its ideal, ultimately, would be to reach not the meaning of words, but the meaning of things themselves. This is why it clouds the language, increases as much as it can the abstractness of the concept and the arbitrariness of the sign and stretches to the limit the link between signifier and signified. . . . This is why our modern poetry always asserts itself as a murder of language, a kind of spatial, legible analogue of silence. (133–34)

I do not here wish to engage the problem of "things in themselves," although this would return us nicely to Stevens (and to Stein) and to the quotes with which I began this paper. I do not wish either to argue at length about why this theoretical agenda seems itself canonical at the moment—it is not self-evident to me that ideological investigations are the natural domain of literary critics and scholars; quite the opposite. What I wish most forcefully to suggest is that Barthes's prose points to a useful analogy between theory and much of contemporary writing: poets are always already theorists and not simply subjects seeking expression of their subjective realities (this is merely our weak notion of what autobiographical poets of preceding generations have been up to).

It is not useful to see poetry as the opposite of theory (like the simplified opposition between Ginsberg and Rich in my example from Martin, such an opposition ensures a conservative interpretation of what poetry is); rather, we must see that contemporary poetry is concerned—and concerned in a theoretical way—with the ontological and epistemological issues that arise when the legitimacy of language is no longer taken for granted. Certainly the recent journalistic drubbing taken by John Ashbery when his *Selected Poems* was issued suggests that the problem of language has not been resolved in our critical thinking (much less that the theorists have won the battle). But the issue I am getting at here is not just the "Ashbery" problem (a problem that for many comes down to "if *I* don't understand him how can I teach him to my students: where is that handy anthology that teaches me how to read his work?"). It is the problem of Rich, Creeley, O'Hara, Plath—all of the writers already "in" our canon; and if it touches all of them differently according to their stake in the cultural systems of gender, class, and race, we need to hand the problem of language to our students as the problem of contemporary poetry and writing; we need to free theory from its place as the unconscious of the curriculum, and that is exactly what it is at the moment—the unconscious, what we will not speak: "Don't say *that* in front of the children! They'll find out about *that* when they're ready!"

Our students are ready; they must be made ready, for they cannot understand what is at stake in contemporary poetry unless they appreciate the current debate about language as a problematic. They need not read Derrida's *Of Grammatology* or Lacan's *Four Fundamental Concepts,* but if they do not see language as a system of differences, if they see it still as a medium for the expression of the poet's agony and insight, then no shake-up in the canon is going to remove them from the tyranny of the great white heterosexual Father and his language. They will still be reading in a phallogocentric fashion. To cite Theodor Adorno: "Your feelings insist that [the lyric] remain [opposed to society], that lyric expression, having escaped from the weight of material existence, evoke the image of a life free from the coercion of reigning practices, of utility, of the relentless pressures of self-preservation.

This demand, however, the demand that the lyric word be virginal, is itself social in nature" (*Notes to Literature* 39). While the handy allusion to "virginity" opens an entire other problematic of sexual difference, modernity, and critical objectivity that we have time only to acknowledge and not to interrogate, the point here is that we need to understand our teaching, reading, and writing of poems, criticism, and theory as part of the material world, as a response to and interrogation of what it means to be a subject in discourse. Writing does not occur outside theory or ideology, and we cannot allow them to be kept outside the debate about or investigation of the canonical.

The Stuttering I: Lyric Subjectivity and Excess

Ich, ich, ich, ich, ich
—Sylvia Plath

To write poetry after Auschwitz is barbaric.
—Theodor Adorno

When we speak of politics and the lyric, a number of possibilities come to mind: one could, on the most mundane level, define as "political" only those poems whose announced theme or interest refers to specific conditions of political or social history: poems like Adrienne Rich's "Rape," or Archibald MacLeish's forgotten texts from the 1930s like *Conquistador,* seem to announce themselves as strictly "political" texts. Or one could read the work of Blake, Shelley, and Byron as an attempt to alter the regime of an Enlightenment they found philosophically and politically repressive: this was how Romanticism was disseminated as revolutionary in my undergraduate days. But a political reading of lyric poetry surely needn't concentrate only on poems that mark their themes as overtly "political." This would have the effect of removing the question of politics from the present reading of the text, making it only a question of historical reference; and it is in the reading of the text that its politics are made, not in the themes or questions it addresses. As Tony Bennett has suggested, "the task which faces Marxist criticism is not that of reflecting or bringing to light the politics which is already there, as a latent presence within the text which has to be made manifest. It is that of actively politicizing the text, of making its politics for it, by producing a new position for it within the field of cultural relations" (167–68).

The most interesting recent political reading of Romanticism, to continue for a moment on that topic, has not been the kind of thematic reading I've mentioned above, but has focused on what Marjorie Levinson calls "the resist[ance to] historical elucidation," on how the representational strategies of Romanticism reduce the political, social, and economic world to a problem in phenomenology and that to a problem in aesthetics, to what even Keats recognized as "the egotistical sublime" (*Wordsworth's Great Period Poems* 55). Its texts are not Wordsworth's sonnets on capital punishment or Toussaint L'Ouverture but *The Prelude*, "Tintern Abbey," "Peele Castle"—the "same" Wordsworth read differently, used to produce a new position for the sign "Wordsworth" in the field of cultural relations. What I am interested in doing with this essay (and I can only hope to point in certain directions) is question the way in which recent poetry in America that announces itself as politically motivated and committed (and my example here will be Robert Lowell) in fact recapitulates to the Romantic disappearance of history in the very act of appearing to do the opposite—*and*, in working against the dominant reading of the "Confessional" poets, collapses lyric subjectivity with personhood and/or personality (my example here will be Sylvia Plath). If we understand that the politics of a text do not reside *in* it as a potential but magically hidden meaning, and rather that its politics are, as are its other "features," produced always in the context of the text's re-production in the anthology, classroom, article, seminar, or individual reading, we should also beware that little has been done to problematize the political act of reading and interpreting poetry *per se* despite the plethora of books and careers recently devoted to political theory and criticism. I would like to spend a moment on this problem before moving on to the specific texts I wish to talk about.

Various critics, including Terry Eagleton, have commented upon Marxism's apparent lack of interest in poetry as a signifying practice, suggesting that it has been easier for Marxist critics to address more transparently social forms like the novel or the drama than to investigate poetry's ideological allegiances. Eagleton has pushed against this tendency, but even revisionary critical projects in American Studies often fail to address poetry as a significant part of their inquiry. The editors of *The American Renaissance Reconsidered,* for instance, whose volume collects representative essays of the New Historicism in American Studies, congratulate themselves on rectifying certain exclusionary mistakes of F. O. Matthiessen's *American Renaissance,* including in their reconsideration of American literature and its political agenda in the nineteenth century: the "sentimental" novelists; Edgar Allen Poe; Frederick Douglass; Harriet Beecher Stowe—all excluded from serious consideration by Matthiessen. But Walter Benn Michaels and Donald Pease neither acknowledge Emily Dickinson's original exclusion from Matthiessen's book nor include her in their own; Walt Whitman is the only poet whose text is discussed at length and he is seen less as a poet and more as an ideologue within the text of American literary history (the distinction I am reaching for here is between Harold Bloom, who reads Whitman as a poet, I think, and someone like R. W. B. Lewis and the myth critics, who do not). Now noncanonical but then highly visible poets like William Cullen Bryant, Robert Lowell, John Greenleaf Whittier, or Henry Wadsworth Longfellow are nowhere reconsidered from this political context that congratulates itself on reconsidering virtually everything else.

The same is true of Sacvan Bercovitch and Myra Jehlen's *Ideology and Classic American Literature.* Both of these works are exemplary as ideological inquiries into the academic study of American culture, but it is remarkable (and symptomatic) that they choose not to consider poetry in a markedly "political" project. If we try to understand why this is, we must confront one more legacy of formalism—the notion that the poem is not referential (in this case "discursively referential") in the same way that fictions, political pamphlets, and dramas are. An influential materialist theory of language and literature such as M. M. Bakhtin's, for instance, makes its claims mostly for fictions and fails to see that poetry may also function as a mode of conflicting social discourses and practices. Surprisingly, some of Bakhtin's essays point directly toward poetry as a "pure" use of language: "The poet is a poet insofar as he accepts the idea of a unitary and singular language, and a unitary, monologically sealed-off utterance" (296–97). Bakhtin does not ordinarily contend that language can escape the social conditions of its own use, production, and exchange; more often he asserts the opposite, and hence we should perhaps read the first statement here as an assertion of the poet's ascription of monologic capacities to language and not as a statement about the actual achievement of a linguistic unity around the intentions of an authorial presence.

Although it has been used by critics to bolster the most conservative uses of literature in our culture, T. S. Eliot's *The Waste Land* in fact exemplifies the radical multiplicity that is social language, constructing itself from an absent center of conflicting voices and cultural discourses. This text is not, of course, strictly lyric, but what we must forego is the notion that the lyric—unlike the epic or narrative poetic text—is, in fact, the record of a single voice; the lyric, like the nonlyric, is multiply crossed by voices and intentions: by ideology. The poet may, as Bakhtin claims, attempt to purify language and make it his or her own, removing the traces of otherness he or she finds there, but this is always only an attempt, and the pressures that fracture fiction and keep it beyond authorial or individual control also fracture the production of poetry and keep it a weave of voices and discourses rather than a single voice, language, or word.

The difference in lyric poetry, and I would claim that there is a difference and that that difference is important (as Dickinson puts it, it is in "the internal difference, / Where the meanings are" ["There's a certain Slant of light"]), is that the lyric is produced in the conventions of subjective unity, in a code that collapses closed meaning and persona, "self." I want to do more here than reiterate notions of the Althusserian "hailing" of the subject; what we need to remember in citing Althusser on interpellation into symbolic discourse is that there is more than one discourse, more than one discursive position, more than one hailing. In a reading of subjectivity that follows a narrow constructionist line, there is no room for resistance—no sense of being able to be Other than what discourse defines. We should remember that Ernesto Laclau repeatedly reminds us that a class is hegemonic not through the imposition of force, but through its ability to neutralize contesting versions of the "real" (see Laclau and Mouffe). The same might be said of discourse. Additionally, we should remember that the subject is always in excess of its hailing, its particular momentary appearance or self-recognition. This is what makes interpellation possible: that there is always something more that exceeds any particular site of subjectivity. The "I" is always elsewhere, that which is not now being discussed. This is the material out of which ideology may put the subject to use. And in the era of commodity aesthetics, it might be better to call this process the "solicitation" rather than the "hailing" of the subject, so that we recall that seduction operates in it, that this process occurs in a libidinal as well as political economy.

The work of the confessionalists (and I like that term because it is so wrong) puts numerous pressures on the conventions of a unified lyric presence in addition to this slippage of the subject, which might be seen in any use of language. (And we should remember that their work is not just autobiographical, and that autobiography is in this instance not just the comfortable home of the colluding bourgeois subject.) What might help us not to read confessionalist work as other than naive subjectivity transparently recorded is a fuller awareness of the pressures against self-knowledge thematized in it: their work is framed, for instance, by a battle between psychoanalysis and psychiatry that is played out across the bodies, lives, and pages of a generation (and in this case, a generation of poets). The conflict I mean to point to here is that between psychiatry's relatively unchallenged institutional power as a science and the more skeptical process of psychoanalysis, which is concerned with the word as a sign of absent or lost desire (Robert Lowell, for instance). Think of being in the remarkably contradictory position of having shock therapy administered to one while being told in therapy that autobiographical investigation was the key to mental health.

In addition, the vogue of existentialism, which Lowell and Plath both use occasionally as a posture and occasionally as a spur to inquire into the "meaning" of a life, the center of which has not held, puts great pressure on the lyric subject and his or her "autobiographical" project. Cold War politics, the bomb, and the inception of a commodified art industry all play their part, too, in the speechlessness that overtakes writers like Plath and Lowell. Reading their work politically means reading against the myths of Lowell and Plath that would make it simple autobiography, and against the larger, framing myths of "confessionalism" that have commodified them in an academic game and reduced their work to bits of information. It is the "I" that stutters its excess, where it cannot be grafted into language, that the confessional poet seeks to represent: the way in which it is misrepresented in the very moment of its representation is his or her focus (I am thinking here of John Berryman in particular, but we can see this in any number of others as well: Theodore Roethke, Anne Sexton, Randall Jarrell, Allen Ginsberg—the subject is endlessly misrepresented by government, psychology, sex, even literature).

What Plath seems to understand is that there is no move to "proper" representation, that there is no way to speak the excess of the "I" except in silence, disfigurement, or visionary madness—that every other position within discourse is merely "set up." Lowell's "madness," on the other hand (and it seldom becomes a textual madness, the madness of writing), is the kind of discomfort that arises from the desire to be rational in an irrational world or irrational body. The very structure of the verse—its interreferentiality (and I do not mean by this its "intertextuality" but its dependence upon motif), its continuous turn to moments of strong closure—each of these turns us away from the possibility that this may be a difficulty we do not yet know how to negotiate or name. What we find in the work of Lowell and Plath, then, if we understand lyric subjectivity as the site of excess, is that in Lowell this excess is always controlled under the figure of the author in search of those terms that will best represent his life, while in Plath there is never any sense of narrative continuity or of the "personal story" granting individual moments their meaning. Despite the clearly autobiographical reference of some of the works, excess is not controlled. Rather, when Plath's poems recount exemplary confrontations with the question of existential meaning, they do so as an encounter with the symbolic: the discourses of masculinity and femininity; of Catholicism, Jewishness (as opposed to Judaism); madness and vision; motherhood; death; mythology—subjectivity in her work is always determined not as a discourse of the "self" but by the crossing of discourses in which any genuine "self" can only be defined through the mechanisms of denial and absence. (Compare Lowell's "Waking in the Blue" [81–82], where "Absence!" is thematized as a complaint of personal loss and recuperated to meaningfulness through literary allusion and balanced motifs, to the process of absence in Plath's "Ariel," where the body moves from "Stasis in darkness" to disintegration, and where enjambment works against even syntactical balance: "And I / Am the arrow, / / The dew that flies / Suicidal, at one with the drive / Into the red / / Eye, the cauldron of morning" [*Ariel* 26–27].)

I would like to turn to Robert Lowell's "Memories of West Street and Lepke," which we might read as an inversion of Wordsworth's "Tintern Abbey." Like the Wordsworth poem, "Lepke" looks backward at a moment in the subject's life that he considers more vital, but unlike it,

"Lepke" focuses on, among other things, that subject's relation to the state (in Wordsworth, this appears only in the dating of the poem; as Marjorie Levinson has written, July 13, the day before Bastille Day, is the unnamed historical catastrophe in the poem ["The New Historicism" 16]). The Lowell poem places its subject at the center of a moral drama, seeking some sense of a genuine subjectivity, a self that, as Walter Benjamin writes of the storyteller, is "the figure in which the righteous man encounters himself" (109). No longer a "fire-breathing Catholic C.O." incarcerated after "telling off the state and president," the speaker has become no better than the other residents on "Boston's / 'hardly passionate Marlborough Street,' / where even the man / scavenging filth in the back alley trash cans, / has two children, a beach wagon, a helpmate, / and is a 'young Republican'" (85). Like this young Republican, he, too, has a "nine months' daughter," who "rises" in her "flame-flamingo infants' wear" (85). (Commodification and the language of advertisement here define even the relation to one's offspring.) "These are the tranquillized *Fifties,*" the text reports, and Lowell turns from them and the sense of diminishment he feels in this larger history to his own personal history, to his moral "seedtime" (a Wordsworthian term straight from "Tintern Abbey") in order to reestablish his moral authority in some economy other than the one in which he "hog[s] a whole house" and "Only teach[es] on Tuesdays" (85). In the final turn to "*Murder Incorporated's* Czar Lepke," we are invited to see both Lowell and his opposite each condemned to isolation among objects "forbidden the common man"—except for Lepke this isolating private property is not his moral stringency and poetic madness, as it is for Lowell, but "a portable radio, a dresser, two toy American / flags tied together with a ribbon of Easter palm" (86).

The play of subjectivity within the person marked "Lowell" throughout *Life Studies* is great: to some extent, its purpose is exactly that of Wordsworth's *Prelude,* to prove (against all evidence) that the subject is a single, cohesive, and integrated being. In "Lepke," the possibly violent disruptions of identity are delimited through construction of an alter ego who signifies secure boundaries between self and Other, past and present, for although these appear ambiguous and slippery, each is ultimately knowable. The major burden of his appearance in the poem seems to be that Lepke, as a synecdoche for American capitalism and its collusion with a "Flabby, bald, lobotomized" (86) Christianity (other inmates have been named Jehovah's Witnesses or speculative, vegetarian metaphysicians), and as a figure who faces "no agonizing reappraisal" (the phrase is John Foster Dulles's description of the Cold War), has no conscience; he functions here to make the conscientious-ness of "Lowell" appear real—and not merely as the property of a leisured middle-class man of letters. What I mean by this is what the middle class discovered in (to look forward to "For the Union Dead") "the last war," that a private conscience is not enough, politically speaking—that the category of "conscientious objector," which was the only way resistance could be officially encoded at first, was insufficient in the face of the fiasco of Vietnam, and that something beyond the individual's private conscientious response was called for.

In "For the Union Dead," placed not merely as the last poem in the dual volume but as the philosophical and moral *telos* of *Life Studies and For the Union Dead,* we see the retreat into quietism and despair that accompany the late Romantic liberalism that marks politics in Lowell: the "savage servility" of Boston (72); the emptiness of the civic project (seen in the pointed contrast between the statue by St. Gaudens commemorating "Colonel Shaw / and his bell-cheeked Negro infantry" [71] from the Civil War and the continuing segregation in American life); the failure of supposedly democratic modes of representation adequately to address searing political issues ("a commercial photograph / shows Hiroshima boiling / over a Mosler Safe, the 'Rock of Ages' / that survived the blast" and on his "television set, / the drained faces of Negro school-children" [72]). Representation fails its own best political intentions (in the St. Gaudens' relief, in the television documentary, in the Lowell poem) because—as the advertisement suggests—the most unthinkable horrors become mere images to be circulated. "For the Union Dead" carries in it a critique of the very means through which Lowell has legitimated his entire career: the image made meaningful by a secure referentiality is no longer available; but the only alternative to this for Lowell is despair, poignancy, a continuing insistence that the personal is there "instead of" the political, that the personalized is the only form in which history takes place.

In turning to the work of Sylvia Plath, we have to ask: how does one read her? That is the question her text keeps asking, not just how can one stand to read it, but also, how, literarily, is one to read it? As prophecy? as autobiography? as death-wish? against the culture that produced it? What makes it difficult to settle this question is that Plath is, in the most radical Emersonian tradition, an un-settler; hers is the kind of writing that decenters meaning, making it happen elsewhere. "Daddy," for instance, opens with the line "You do not do, you do not do," and offers as a moment in counterpoint the lyric subject's ironic marriage to its destructive Other, written in the phrase: "I do, I do" (*Ariel* 49). But the signifier of Otherness in this text is most dramatically "German," in its famous image of Nazis, and in Plath's extraordinary stuttering of herself in the following lines: "I never could talk to you. / The tongue stuck in my jaw. / It stuck in a barb wire snare. / Ich, ich, ich, ich" (*Ariel* 49). But surely this play of pronouns across two languages takes us back to the "do-ing" that fills the text as well, and we recognize that this is also a "du"-ing, an "Ach, du," a familiar Other in which one recognizes one's place as an "ich." The subject here is quite literally a signifier for another signifier, and each of these exceeds the meaning of its pronominal reference. It is in such language that Plath sees the staging of the patriarchal control of subjectivity, and "Daddy" is only the most egregious example of the critique of patriarchal Otherness seen everywhere in her work.

Any reading that equates the poem's "Daddy" with a biological or autobiographical father explains the poem without reference to the discourses through which it takes up the question of female subjectivity annihilated by patriarchal injunctions against it. Adorno wrote "To write poetry after Auschwitz is barbaric" (*Prisms* 34269), and I apologize for the ease with which one may invoke Auschwitz since it is so difficult actually to say anything about it—indeed, it is a sign for what is unspeakable about our era. But this is one way to think about the destructive poetics of Sylvia Plath: that "poetry after Auschwitz" indeed has to be barbaric itself in order to avoid capitulation to the very principles that produced the Holocaust; it must be a barbaric rather than a "meaningful" or civilized project. This is how I think we might read her turn to violent images: not as the morbid response of an unstable ego but as the political response of a decivilized one. In the work of Sylvia Plath we see something like a pointed protest against the cultural hegemonies imposed on women— as Lowell writes in his introduction to *Ariel,* the figural subject at the center of Plath's lyrics is "one of those super-real, hypnotic, great classical heroines" (vii). But the question he never takes up is what happens when a woman finally assumes this role as opposed to merely reciting lines from Racine or Shakespeare? What happens is anger, violence that can only be sanctioned as self-destruction, the need to destroy the body, to become a "pure acetylene / Virgin / Attended by . . . / whatever these pink things mean," rising "To Paradise" (*Ariel* 54–55).

But even in this poem of delirium, with its revision of Dickinson's "possibility" at its close, as her "selves dissolv[e], old whore petticoats" (55), it is the discourse that does the work: all ironic, the Christian drive for a purified woman, the poetic drive for a saintly one, the notion that the female body is always already enclosed by its own whoredom, that the female self has been bought and sold: this is not experience, this is the deployment of meaning through a cultural semiotics so dense that there is no subjectivity undefined by its power, no self except what can be annihilated in language. I have only a few moments to glance at the poem "Edge," where the lyric subject revises Medea:

> The woman is perfected.
> Her dead
>
> Body wears the smile of accomplishment,
> The illusion of a Greek necessity
>
> Flows in the scrolls of her toga,
> Her bare
>
> Feet seem to be saying:
> We have come so far, it is over.
>
> Each dead child coiled, a white serpent,
> One at each little
>
> Pitcher of milk, now empty.
> She has folded
>
> Them back into her body as petals
> Of a rose close when the garden
>
> Stiffens and odours bleed
> From the sweet, deep throats of the night flower.
>
> The moon has nothing to be sad about,
> Staring from her hood of bone.
>
> She is used to this sort of thing.
> Her blacks crackle and drag.
> (*Ariel* 84)

This is a sure reversal of standard tropes and discourses signifying "woman"—motherhood, the garden, the moon, a perfect body, and the most pointed of all: the refusal of sentimentality or poignancy.

What we see in Plath is the desire to articulate a vision whose antagonism is not immediately neutralized. This is, I would claim, a political poetry, and occurs even when the poems are not thematically "about" politics—*and,* and this is more surprising, given the years in which these were written, even when they turn pointedly away from history toward a problem of the symbolic. Plath's claim on our attention is that her poetry never grounds its excess in any familiarizing referentiality, but makes its lyric subject stutter always toward some thing it knows but cannot say. (Even our past notions of feminism fail at times, since hers is not a text of "active resistance" but of representational guerrilla warfare.) Her poetry is always concerned with what it cannot articulate; that is the "edge" it cuts. From "The Colossus," the title-poem to her first volume:

> I shall never get you put together entirely,
> Pieced, glued, and properly jointed.
>
> Perhaps you consider yourself an oracle,
> Mouthpiece of the dead, or of some god or other.
> Thirty years now I have labored
> To dredge the silt from your throat.
> I am none the wiser.
>
> .   .   .   .   .
>
> Nights, I squat in the cornucopia
> Of your left ear, out of the wind,
>
> Counting the red stars and those of plum-color.
> The sun rises under the pillar of your tongue,
> My hours are married to shadow.
> No longer do I listen for the scrape of a keel
> On the blank stones of the landing.
> (*The Colossus* 20–21)

This is the poetry of a resistance we have only begun to know. We do not have a politics of the lyric until it takes this poetry into account.

The Mortal Limits of Poetry and Criticism:
Reading Yingling, Reading Gunn

Robert L. Caserio

The acid trip is unstructured, it opens you up to countless possibilities, you hanker after the infinite. The only way I could give myself any control over the presentation of these experiences and so could be true to them, was by trying to render the infinite through the finite.—Thom Gunn, 1979

The attractiveness and the distinction of the late Thomas Yingling's *Hart Crane and the Homosexual Text* derives from Yingling's performance of multiple, indeed self-divided, and even self-contradictory, critical intentions. On the one hand, Yingling's book opposes the transcendental and universalizing impulse in Crane's poetry, and insists on returning the poet's opaque flights of sublimity to the specific situatedness of Crane's psyche and of his historical time and place. Simultaneously, on the other hand, Yingling's book, in spite of its love for historical specificity, endorses a sublime universal of its own: diacritics, writing, the global textual nature of desire and of the world. But there are critics, I submit, in whom self-contradiction enables a tem-

peramental and intellectual generosity toward their objects, and a capacity for fine analysis of them, in comparison with which a more
rigorous critical coherence is disabling and cold. I count Yingling high
among critics empowered by their internal divisions. How these divisions operate, and how they articulate a critical and artistic moral for
our moment, is best spelled out in the relation of Yingling's book to its
subject's mortality.

Yingling represents Crane's suicide as the product of America's hatred of homosexuality and of Crane's misprision of the true, purely
textual or diacritical, being of both eros and language. Amounting to a
critical therapy for Crane's willful embrace of death, the critic's work
tries to rescue Crane from suicide, and from the causes that drove
Crane toward it. Yet the rescue attempt shows the critic's self-division
already in play. For Yingling, Crane's death certifies the intransigence
and integrity of the poet's homosexuality. In spite of homophobia,
Crane's desire triumphs in death, using mortality to stop the limitless
play of diacritical differences, to make a fixed stand on behalf of a
determinate homosexual desire. Crane, figured by the critic on one
page as the agent of a "cruelly disabling and isolating vision of homosexuality" (Yingling 189) can be refigured, within the space of a few
pages, as the agent of "a reclamation of homosexuality and the body as
well" (193). Consider, for a further example of the critic's analytic self-
division, Yingling's rhetoric as he estimates the success of Crane's "Repose of Rivers": "[I]f [Crane's] life had by the summer of 1926 *already
become a plague from which he could not escape* . . . the poem nevertheless bravely signals [his] refusal to surrender his project for homosexual centrality. . . . Crane's lyrics, . . . *it is not hyperbolic to say, at the
cost of his life* . . . allow homosexual subjectivity to be heard as *authentic experience*" (144; emphasis added). In this way of putting it, the
poet's life is the long disease of American homophobia; and the life
begins to mend when, matched with the poet's integrity in standing
true to his experience and desire, self-elected death brings Crane all
the vital things he wanted from both his sexual and his poetic callings.

Nevertheless, while the critic pictures Crane's life as a death from
which his mortal demise was a poetic rebirth of life, the critic has other
ways of picturing the phenomenon. He prefers the other ways. In what
I've described, the close mingling of life and death in Crane, their
phoenixlike incarnation of each other, suggests a phenomenology or
even an ontology that Yingling decidedly distrusts. While tracing
Crane's contradictions, Yingling does not appear to want his critical

stance to be their replica. He trusts instead in his intellectual commitment to a consistent and all-unifying claim that life and death,
homosexuality and heterosexuality, and all the contrasts and differences or all the similarities that we can name, are not substances or
identities or realities, whether delimited or intermingled; they are
words and texts, rather, infinitely in process and discursive. How does
Yingling most intend to save "Repose of Rivers" from its author's (and
its own) besetting mortality? He does so by moving, rather like the
poem, from what seems specific and delimited to what is less so. He
designates a specification or limitation of experience or meaning in the
poem only to move beyond, up onto the peak of a theoretical and
sublime semiosis. Although Yingling admits, to begin with, that in
"Repose of Rivers" "the homosexual text," as he puts it (already he
signals homosexuality not as a definite practice but as an open discourse), is "obscure," he declares, in spite of the obscurity, that it is
"right to read [the poem] as a text of homosexual authorization" (139).
He declares this in order to allegorize the poem as "a model of homosexual subjectivity that moves beyond . . . family romance and its strict
duality of masculine and feminine identities" (139). Significantly, the
allegorization moves not only beyond these strict dual identities, but
beyond homosexual identity as well. Designating "Repose of Rivers"'s
climactic audition of wind flaking sapphire as a figure of homosexual
inspiration, the critic—to judge from what he says earlier about Crane's
"Voyages"—also must hear the sound as the inspiration of language
understood "not as a medium of incarnation" (103), and not as a medium of identification, but as one of resounding "difference, of diacritics, of writings" (103). Homosexual authenticity is not found in bodily
sexual practice, or in identity, but in one sole "authenticity": diacritics. The enfranchisement of homosexuality takes place out on the limitless ocean that is language, blown upon by the boundless winds of
words. On the freedom of the seas of difference, the critic rescues the
poet's drowned body and desire from the limitations of the conventionally identifiable, literal, and fatal ocean. The means of rescue from
mortality is theory. In the liberty of theory, moreover, rather than in
homosexuality "per se," there is the approximate realization of "the
unmarried epic" and "the homosexual sublime," the phrases whereby
Yingling names the objects of Crane's baffled quest.

   The sea of textual differences serves many life-saving purposes
in Yingling's analysis. It is the point of repair from narrow and life-
threatening false distinctions and oppositions in which Crane is said

by the critic (unlike the critic?) to be invested: a false division between poetic universality and historical specificity; a falsely straitening opposition of homosexual love to all other love; a false distinction between mind and (homosexual) body. When, in a spirit said by Yingling to be antithetical to "Repose of Rivers," Crane wrote "The Broken Tower," the writing was the prophecy of his suicide, for according to Yingling "The Broken Tower" gives way to Crane's conviction that homosexuality is a failure of life, because it cannot become the "pure being" (182) a punitive patriarchal Other demands that it be. In "The Broken Tower," we are told, the poet tragically loses his nerve to live in the inevitable allegory that is language and desire. Accordingly, Yingling says, "The Broken Tower" is a text in which "autobiography becomes an act of death" (185), for life is eternal allegoresis, according to the critic; whereas death is simply the end.

It is here, however, in the attempt to construct out of a theory of diacritics a realm of vitality and homosexuality safe from death, that Yingling's contradictions poignantly show through. Yingling's picture of Crane's willful wandering into death designates modernist poetics's supposedly mistaken idea about language as the crucial instrument of Crane's self-destructive error. The assumption of *Hart Crane and the Homosexual Text* is that modernist poetics amounts to a stubbornly wrong attempt to displace language in two erroneous directions, toward two impossible "places": toward a mystifying, language-transcending reference point; toward illusive limitary incarnations (the word made flesh) and determinate, fixed moments of being or meaning. The critic insists that Crane might have overcome his errors by a more proper address to displacement. The more proper form is poststructuralist: it avoids language's illusive tendencies; it recognizes the unlimited character of signification, albeit without mystifying the infinity of discourse. Still and all, the question arises: how can one tell what is proper from what's improper? The critic, even as he discriminates good forms of displacement from bad, himself gives in to uses of the bad kind. Crane's death, used by the critic as a limitary fact, dictates, delimits Yingling's interpretation of "The Broken Tower," so that the poem *must* be identified as an unbridgeable contrast with "Repose of Rivers," as the seal of Crane's death—his very suicide. And yet "Repose of Rivers," whose mode of modernist linguistic displacement makes its status as authentically homosexual text uncertain and obscure, as the critic admits, is read by Yingling simultaneously (and self-contradictorily) as if a transparently clear homosexual writing and a transparently identifiable homosexual being shine through the obscurity. But the critic's improper displacement, it turns out, enables a brilliant reading; just as Crane's improper displacement of language produces brilliant poems. Limitation, an inhibition of restless diacritics, distance from safety, and closeness to death are not (after all) the enemies of life.

Now in making these demurrers my intention is not to mortify Yingling, whose loss to me remains personally and intellectually wrenching. It had been my intention to propose and debate these contradictions with Yingling in life. I trust he would have allowed and welcomed the debate, on the basis of an exchange of letters I had begun with him in 1991, as well as on the basis of another facet of *Hart Crane and the Homosexual Text,* one that strikes me as the real reason for the theory there, a basis that the theory makes possible, but is separable from. Indeed it is the theory in Yingling's criticism that I think is mortal and that I propose does not possess the secure vitality we all have trusted for so long in doing our collective work. What is more secure and vital than theory in Yingling, what makes one (I hope) generously note the contradictions inherent in his trust in the diacritical life-line, is an alternative strategy: his attempt to use his book to recreate himself as Crane's advocate and other self. The theory in Yingling functions like a Yeatsian mask, for the purpose of getting the personal man in place. And the person under the critical persona is a Yingling-Crane, whose especial source is Crane's feisty letters, the ones in which—beginning when he is nineteen years old, when he reveals to Gorham Munson that the object of a recent love affair is not a *her,* but a *him*—Crane stands up, now plainly, now giddily and extravagantly, against homophobic pressure to hide the nature of his eros. Although Yingling actually criticizes the extravagance, in a curious extension of homophobic hurt; indeed, although Yingling rebukes Crane for misunderstanding and misusing the sublime freedoms of the diacritical universe, he nevertheless situates himself both as the writer of Crane's last letter to his culture, and as still Crane's friend—a critic-lover-friend, the one friend and lover who does not abandon Crane even as he criticizes him.

Hart Crane and the Homosexual Text is subliminally but most powerfully a correspondence with Crane; the accompanying theory, the necessary envelope and postmark. The book on Crane gives us a critic whose reading of his subject's way of loving is simultaneously the defense of the critic's own way, and is therefore the projection of a same-sex love affair into the living space in which the critic evokes his poet. While such love affairs, whether "hetero" or "homo," are likely to be always the stuff of criticism, it is notable how often the erotic link is buried or anesthetized in the current deployment of "theory," even the queerest. Queer theory's logically faultless subversion of homosexual "identity" has tended, ironically, to put eros at a distance from critics' efforts to recapture it. The irony is tellingly described in James Creech's *Closet Writing/Gay Reading.* In Yingling the contradictions at the level of theory, forecasting the state of critical affairs described by Creech, seem the signs of a palpable personal love at work. For, after all, what characterizes the critic's love is fixation, the intellectual equivalent of the dogged devotion of an erotic commitment, which in its repeated stress on keeping both the beloved and love in existence, is far more limited, limiting, and unfree than the limitless textuality the devotion is alleged to approximate. Finiteness of attachment, circumscription of focus, an involuntary self-limiting, are observable characteristics of eros. Our will to free homosexuality from fetters is I think our aim, as much as anything, to respect and dignify the non-idealizing, non-infinitizing characteristics of all sexual love. We free, paradoxically, the power of erotic constraint over us. In Crane, one should notice, every expansion of meaning is always pulled back into the narrows of formal control: precisely the tension, the pressure of constraint upon inspiration and sex gives Crane's poetry its characteristic difficulty *and* its characteristic eroticism. The source of Yingling's expansive theory is the same tension between the limitlessness of the realm of theory and the fixated, limitary, eroticized attachment at its heart.

In drawing a line from Yingling to Creech, I've already hinted at the way *Hart Crane and the Homosexual Text* in retrospect appears to have predicted current developing—and divided—intellectual trajectories in queer cultural studies. The intellectual force of Lee Edelman's *Homographesis* shows the still-vivid power of the poststructuralist mode that was Yingling's most conscious inspiration. Yet alternative inspirations in his study of Crane—the enacted valuation of something that is more personal and modest than "theory," of something no less submissive to history and fate than rebellious against them—predicts the emphases of such recent work as Teresa de Lauretis's *The Practice of Love* and Leo Bersani's *Homos.* The title of de Lauretis's book insists, after all, that the consummation of theory's flights must take place on the more limited ground of practice; it is no accident, moreover, that

the insistence accompanies the critic's attempt to model lesbian practices on fetishism—on, that is, an erotic form of constraining fixation.
And Bersani's brilliant summing up of queer theory's fortunes ends
with a celebration, apropos of Jean Genet's *Funeral Rites,* of homoerotic wastefulness, of homosexuality's refusal of productive and re-
productive duties; in short, of its closeness to mortality. The tension
in Yingling's book between allegiance to the limitlessness of theory
and the limitariness of eros is one essential origin of present critical
debates.

For putting things in this way about the development of criticism,
my authority is not queer theory per se, however. My authority is neither "theory" nor "literary criticism," but poetry (the supreme theory,
arguably). I would have tried to persuade Yingling that my reading of
his self-divided dynamics is not unjust, that it has some corrobora-
tion in contemporary gay *poetics,* by having asked him to meditate
on Thom Gunn's *Jack Straw's Castle* and *The Passages of Joy* (both
pre-AIDS volumes) as well as on *The Man with Night Sweats.* My re-
quest would have fully acknowledged, to begin with, the explicit presence in Gunn's poems of the poet's poststructuralist consciousness of
the textuality of his realm. The much-cited poem "The Menace," for
example, which is about the threatening aspects of sex between leath-
ermen, proposes—with the help of an embedded excerpt from Gregory
Bateson's writing on playful, "textualizing" displacements of denota-
tion—that a semiotized eros can use play to liberate a fetishized homoerotic maleness from, as the poem says, the strenuous dullness of its
limitations (Gunn 340). Yet what is finally remarkable about Gunn's
poem is that its expansive diacritical play with menace, which would
appear to push back the border of death by expanding this semiosis
that is life, contracts, and returns the homosexual players to limitation.
And the return is curiously blessed, as if the play—in spite of its transformative value—had been an exercise in the personal, loving submis-
sion to the limits rather than the expansive opportunities of sexual
love. Whereas in *Hart Crane and the Homosexual Text* the critic's
appeal to the limiting specificity of historical and cultural situations is
only a moment in a movement toward an unfixed expansion of textuality, in Gunn what is unfixed is only a moment in an opposite
direction. Already in his earlier poems Gunn lays the groundwork for
the way in which *The Man with Night Sweats* takes on power from
pathos: the pathos of homosexuality and friendship working as a form
of mortal limitation, mortified by inherent constraints on loving and

living even as they acknowledge the new twist in mortification produced by the present American moment of history and disease. Yingling's impulsive, nontheoretical doubling of Crane and loving of him parallels Gunn's picture of the intimate, mutually limiting stress that eros, life, and death place upon each other—a stress that makes it difficult to designate life, love, and death as widely contrasting realms, in the way attempted by Yingling's more deliberate aims, dazzled as they are by the unavowed idealizing and infinitizing of life by theory.

Gunn's model for the narrowing of the difference between life's and love's expansiveness, especially in the forms of critical-semiotic speculation and of poetry, and life's and love's limitation (no matter what historical specifics contextualize the limitation), is given more centrally than in "The Menace" in another poem from *The Passages of Joy*, "The Exercise" (331–32). Like "The Menace," "The Exercise" is a conditioning poem; an uncanny rehearsal of habits useful for learning the stress of the new historical limits that are endured in *The Man with Night Sweats*. The speaker of "The Exercise," caught up in a transaction among the weather, a suburban landscape, and poetic inspiration, says "Though the wind was like / impulse, it was not impulse. / If I was formed by it, I was formed / by the exercise it gave me. / Exercise in stance, and / in the muscle of feeling. / I became robust standing against it" (332). Robust health is celebrated in the poem, but the development of strength even in the pre-AIDS era turns out to have its own frailty: for one thing the development is painfully slow. Although the wind is a figure for "the swiftly changing" (332), what the wind plays on is slowly changing. Inspirations, however invigorating, are also mortifying, tardy in turning into endurance or grace. And the grace of endurance is inseparable from one's enduring limits. The exercise—whether of breathing or writing—is, to be sure, a glad one, and tingles, the poem says, "with knowledge" (332); but the path of gladness and knowledge is a narrow passage.

The Man with Night Sweats traces the narrow passage shared by the advance of life and homosexuality and the advance of death in our historical present. In doing so, it several times echoes Crane's "Repose of Rivers," and so furnishes thoughts about Yingling with a relevant endpoint. Gunn's "To a Friend in Time of Trouble" depicts its addressee taking refuge from a plagued city in weekend country labors (408–9). Chores, and climbing, suddenly loose the friend's mind from grief and rage: life returns in the access of release. But is release expansion, the slipping of limits? The poem concludes by saying that "the released mind" . . . "feels the healing start, and still returns, / Riding its own repose, and learns, and learns" (409). The "and learns, and learns" strikes one at first as a form of expansion—and as a form too of trailing off. But when one rereads the apparently *morendo* phrase as instead the syntax of intensification, the impression of both expansion and a slack unwinding is reversed. "And learns, and learns" figures concentration—release and repose are the result of lessons deepening under a delimiting impact. Is the learning not learning to lose as well as to be loosed? Learning and losing, loss and release come together; they are not differentiated or singly sublimed; instead, involved, they repose on mortality. This poem, recollecting its origins in homosexual eros, in mortality and in Crane, hugs all three, characterizing life and homosexuality as a constant nonhomophobic reposing upon one or another vivid limitation. In another echo of "Repose of Rivers," "A Sketch of the Great Dejection," a drearily sublime marsh and ocean are ironically inspiring: "My body insisted on restlessness / having been promised love, / as my mind insisted on words / having been promised the imagination" (Gunn 424). The confluence of these lines is with Yingling even more than with Crane, for Gunn's speaker here settles for restlessness and mere words, and surrenders the desire for incarnation and transcendence, as Yingling repeatedly claims Crane should have done. But a contrast with Yingling also shows itself. Gunn's speaker admits that the fruit of his surrenders is an alertness due to confusion and discomfort. It is not due to what Yingling suggests is the more clear-sighted and more comfortingly expansive result of the diacritics that are said to be more liberating than love. Contradicting this claim, the speakers of Gunn's latest poems repose not on expansiveness but on plainness ("Death is so plain!" [475], the poem "Her Pet" cries out) and painful constraint. In the spirit of "The Exercise," the artist in "Her Pet" makes art out of "A strength so lavish she can limit it" (475). Yet it is hard to tell the strength of this art, however lavish, apart from its limitations, which become its shaping and loving medium.

If there is a contrast between Gunn's and Yingling's aesthetic, erotic, and ethical values, it is only in relation to one aspect of Yingling's makeup: the aspect of the theorist, for whom the theory of discourse is a bulwark against loss and extermination. Is there in this bulwark an echo of heterosexuality's persistent fantasy of love's generative infinity, of unending offspring? But there is, I repeat, another Yingling, the personal lover-shadow of Crane, bare of theory. Yingling's later writings show a Gunn-like dignity, in which the critic is exercised by the stress of adversity, and labors with pain, like the protagonist of "Her Pet," "to bring on its end" (475). In the course of the labor, curiously, a new aesthetic interest emerges; for example, in this posthumous collection's reading of Niedecker and Plath. In them, Yingling points out "the poetry of a resistance we have only begun to know" (157; this volume) and "an aesthetic that challenges the reader in a way foreign to many . . . overtly 'political' . . . texts" (139; this volume). Although political in significance, the resistance and the challenges at issue are achieved, it appears, by an ascesis of the strength of politics and of theory. Their strength is so lavish that now, for the critic, it can repose on, and limit itself to, poetry alone. In these final expressions of his own pained concentration or repose, Yingling is true, in I venture to say a truly homosexual way, to the mortal limits of love, of criticism, and of contemporary art.

Something

When I am silent
I imagine deep meaning,
my skin gone suddenly
away from me—into
some further sense
I cannot follow
but with words
that sound out the flesh.

I have become skeptical
of motives, paranoid perhaps:
this child who once
took his intuitions as a rule.

Creature comforts.
—Figure it.
Include in that
the smiles and hallelujahs,

what was lost before was born:
the names of many, the place
to be, the aching-after care.

Wellness hollows us
but we are unprepared.
Water rises in the hollow.

It is that errancy I seek
within myself: to turn and find
the world was really there.

Caesura

Stephen Melville

Parting, Words

This essay began as a contribution to an MLA panel honoring the memory of Tom Yingling, and attempted to do so by pursuing questions about what AIDS might have to teach us about imaginations of criticism and community. To this question, I wanted to answer (and still do want to answer): nothing. As will become quickly apparent I both do and do not mean this absolutely. What there is to be learned from AIDS is that we die—but this is hardly the "new knowledge" contemporary theory so loves—nor is it clear that it is news to say, as I will, that there is neither criticism nor community apart from this.

A colleague dies, too young; and that dying has the structure of a sentence, so it is a death not simply premature but also prematurely inhabited. This is and is not the common lot, a singular death, like all deaths; and like all deaths, like each death, it recalls—can recall—the common human exposure to death and to one another. Beyond such bare facts there appears to stretch only the vast gray ground of cliché—"a stereotype block," says the OED: words whose linkage is automatic and whose inner articulation has been lost. Clichéd phrases, variously mumbled, inscribed, or withheld (either in denial or out of respect for what cannot be said)—are those through which something, at once a life and a death—something that definitively escapes its survivors—can nonetheless be acceded to. These phrases and the various genres of eulogy, lament, and apostrophe into which they open do not matter, finally, for their work of representation but for something else, something it is tempting to subsume under the linguist's category of phatic communion, a certain gathering together around an emptiness both semantic and real. These phrases appear as if tokens of a ritual order for which a faith is admittedly lacking; and so also they offer a way of overcoming a certain modern speechlessness before death, a speechlessness that may itself appear as if a symptom of a fall from the grace of some more vital tradition or community.

Within modernity, "criticism" frequently enough figures as a name either for that fall or for its causes; it is that thing before whose relentless judgment all received forms, traditions, and communities are asked to stand or fall—and I suppose that is reason enough for the strange repercussions arcane curricular debates can seem to have upon the moral fiber of a nation with its own deep stakes in and confusions about the kind of community it is or is not, wants to be, or does not want to be. But criticism has, of course, also been figured as one of the strongest bulwarks against that fall, as a mode of care for and prolongation of those values that modernity itself ceaselessly undoes, and one can come to care deeply that the forms of criticism as a mode of apparent communion remain intact regardless of one's actual stake or interest in the culture it presumably preserves and passes on.

This second figure opens one way of linking together the terms that entitled the MLA panel. What they finally add up to is a view in which what is to be learned from AIDS is the terms of membership in the human—which is to say mortal, moral, and cultural—community, the terms of what would then be our mutual belonging and legacy. These terms, this nexus of terms above all, sketch out the familiar outline of a mode of thought of which the academic critical community, increasingly given over to criticism in the first sense, has become justly and sustainedly suspicious in recent years. So the question would now be about how a community defined by its relation to criticism—if community it is—can find a way to acknowledge a debt to something called "the human" and evidently inscribed within its practice, while continuing to mark or measure a certain distance from the terms that appear to ground it and the phatic reassurances it offers. In what ways can one speak of the legacies—real or metaphorical, moral or material—that one may feel or find oneself asked to bear?

Out, Living

It is a familiar thought that modernity is marked and worked by a special relation to death: Descartes's withdrawal from the world in order to find its proof can be imagined as a form of suicide, a way of thinking the world on the ground of the thinker's absence from it or of its absence from him—and not simply because he stuck his head in an oven. And Kant's massive critical effort to establish the grounds of possibility for the world or worlds in which we know and act can appear—as it does in Jay Bernstein's *The Fate of Art*—as an extraordinary act of melancholic mourning.

In the nearer past, there have been efforts by Robert Jay Lifton and others to suggest that the postwar generation is well understood as a generation of people who defined themselves as survivors of a sort. The thought as I recall it was that the effect of the ongoing fact and presence of "the bomb" made the world one that had in principle ended—that is, made the world something whose catastrophe had been survived and that was thus inhabited only posthumously. In its moment—the late sixties and early seventies—this thought seemed to connect in multiple ways with such things as Leon Festinger's theories of "cognitive dissonance"—especially as evidenced in the sometimes peculiar, often chiliastic, reactions of those on the fringes of certain disasters, not actually affected by them but close enough to be unable to imagine them simply as someone else's—thus unable either to take such events on for themselves or to set them aside, unable to determine the terms of their inhabitation of that world.

Whatever fascination such notions might once have held for students of culture appears to have receded now behind the wash of theory. And yet they remain interesting descriptions and are perhaps usefully recalled as a part of the background against which current concerns and practices can be figured and which occasionally resurface through them, as for example in the effort to think "the nuclear sublime." More generally, one might note the extent to which a certain rhetoric of survival has penetrated both academic discourse and popular culture—both in those theoretical positions that embrace the description of one's victimization—of what one has survived—as a mode of empowerment and in those ever-burgeoning bookstore sections devoted to "recovery" (as if life itself were increasingly lived as damage survived, at once clung to and surmounted). And then too, of course, there is all our ongoing intrigue with things "post-"—whether we take this up theoretically in terms of "posthistoire," "postaesthetics," "postmodernity," and so on, or in the popular terms proposed by Mad Max, Bill and Ted, *Neuromancer,* and all the movies and fictions that stretch more or less between them. These too have, of course, their own philosophic background, particularly in that bundle of Hegelian claims that seem to amount to an assertion of something like the end of the world.

At a certain level, AIDS seems to repeat or renew all this; it is hardly surprising that the genres of popular culture that have been able to powerfully figure our postapocalyptic situation have shown themselves able to figure AIDS as well. Like Lifton's bomb, it announces a death within the horizon of which one must live, and like the bomb it shifts "survival" away from the disaster, which cannot be survived, to those who live not in it but in its light. The disaster it poses cannot be one's own in that it cannot be survived in the first person; no one, thus far, has been able to escape the wreckage once drawn into it.

But there are, of course, differences as well: the bomb's threat is universal extinction and that extinction is, in imagination if not in fact, immediate. AIDS comes one at a time and its work is not immediate; it comes in the form of a sentence, holding its sufferers in a peculiar pause or parenthesis like the one given powerful expression by Maurice Blanchot's crucially ambiguous "arret de mort," a cusp or ridge in which the end that is death and the suspension of that end are bound together. And it is, of course, from Blanchot that I have taken the term "disaster" as well. One of Jacques Derrida's readings of Blanchot's *recit* unfolds under the title "Survivre," and, like these remarks, it explores a certain disruption of the lines between life and death, between surviving the disaster because one has lived through it and surviving it because one has not. I do not propose to chart all the ways living, living on, and living through can be knotted or unraveled, even in a sentence as simple as the one I've just written: what the fabric itself everywhere displays is at once the absoluteness and finality of the distinction between life and death and the constant passage of the one into and out of the other.

Would it be too much to say that modernity's peculiar orientation to death, to mourning and to living on, has at its heart a certain dream of immunity and immortality, an imagination of the living dead who, because at once living and dead, absolutely attached to their own disaster, hold themselves beyond the grasp of either life or death? And if this is not too much, would it be just to say that this is lived with a particular depth or passion by those who call themselves Americans? Such questions are doubtless too large and too shapeless to permit of serious answering—or perhaps it is America that has become too large or shapeless for their serious posing—although I persist in thinking that something of its myth remains active in the shapes of thought and action I am trying to bring into view—and about which it is perhaps time to come clean.

The thought, derived in part from Stanley Cavell and in part from various French philosophers (Blanchot, Derrida, and Nancy, above all), is just that what one might call the contemporary critical community is everywhere worked by an extraordinary, radical, and self-certifying skepticism that is not without its roots in the broader forms of life within which it finds itself. This skepticism is extraordinary and radical in that it is more fully lived than thought, and it is self-certifying in that it turns inside a confusion or conflation of life and death that finds its fulfillment in a fantasy of immortality rather than in an acknowledgment of mortality and finitude. As a social theory it plays out in a fantasy in which the mutual attachment of damage and identity figured as survival is taken as adequate to the articulation of a social order that can secure, in melancholic recreation, the vanished mythic goods of "community."

Against this, it would be urgent to say that the ever-open passage between life and death such fantasy both draws upon and denies can only ever open toward finitude, can only ever work as exposure to a death that is neither one's own nor appropriable to one's self but which is permanently that of the other. So the nothing to be learned from AIDS is the real nothing that is one's exposure not to what one survives or can imagine one's self to survive, but to him or her whom one outlives. Learning this nothing would be learning to mourn not as a defense against death and absence but as an affirmation of one's exposure to it as continuous with one's essential openness to the other.

The other is then him or her whom you outlive, with and without whom you live out your days, and this outliving is not accidental but structural—that is to say, it is what it is that there are others. To imagine surviving apart from those you outlive and with whom you are lived out is to imagine a world in which there are no others—even if your imagination is that you are not alone but surrounded by those who have survived with you. It is a dark dream of posthumous intimacy freed of all distance, freed of the demand for acknowledgment, freed of separation because locked within it.

Separation is the inescapable condition of community, and there is no greater community to be imagined beyond it: the only question is whether and how that condition is to be acknowledged or denied, how one is to admit or refuse the dispersal of ends and the mutual exposure that is all there is of binding in it. Separation—singularity, as Nancy puts it—is indefeasible, either to be begun from or else to return upon, and against, those imaginations and communities that would turn from it.

Departments, Of Literature

I do not, now, expect to find myself in my teaching and writing apart from someone—colleague, friend, or subject of my scholarly concern—dying too soon. I don't know that this is a new fact in the university, although it is certainly a very old one, so if there has been a certain absence or abeyance it has taken the form of a permission to forget, and the time of that permission has, all things considered, been exceedingly short. It is tempting to say that this time of absence or abeyance is also the time of the self-forgetting of criticism.

There is in the professional critical community (by this I suppose I mean a community that imagines the lives within it taking the shape of careers rather than the shape of a constant exposure to dying)—there is in this community a measuring, a habit of measuring, what is living and what is dead in another's thought or writing as if that were a way of dating it, determining one's distance from it, and of negotiating each time anew the passage from death to life (bringing, then, a voice, a poem, a work to life). This is a deep and persistent habit: if the humanist terms in which I have cast it now seem alien or outmoded, it is far from clear that the current tendency to cast such negotiations in more overtly political terms offers any serious break with them or with the rage against time and separation they represent. These ways of imagining oneself to speak for a community or a tradition conceal an imagination of oneself as immortal or outside the world, thus attempting to turn separation into a trope of belonging and radical inclusion. The work of criticism and of reading—of acknowledging one's exposure to what is other—is the refusal of all such imaginations. It is a way of displaying that interlacing of life and death in the midst of which—by which—what there is of actual community is worked and unworked, rhythmed and sprung. Legacy, thought within the structure of filiation proper to criticism, is neither recovery nor preservation but prolongation of what is always already and only in separation, the thing Blanchot calls a "work" and can describe only in its unworking, its *desouevrement.* This would be the shape of solidarity, in time or in community; it would also be why it matters to think as Blanchot does about the death of the author and the life of the work, about what it means that there are objects that can be only as objects of reading, submitted to a scansion in which they do not return to themselves. And it would be why it matters to be able to read, as Derrida does, a text like *Beyond the Pleasure Principle* as a doing and undoing of legacy, an imagination and denial—an institution—of community.

I do not know why historically we have come to call the elements of our institutions "departments" or "divisions." What I have come to hear in the names of those departments that cannot find their ground in calculation, application, and the simple transmission of knowledge is a movement no curriculum can contain, a movement even in its origins already ruinous or exuberant: aneconomic, mortal, exposed.

AIDS, Community

And have I, in saying all this, said anything about AIDS? I suppose not, so there is perhaps this to be added:

If death came simply from the outside, as perhaps it does for plants and animals (or at least those animals who have not found themselves taken up into and transformed by the terms of human community), it would be a very different thing, unable to support either ritual or politics. But death is in the world as its limit, as the fact of an outside that cannot be touched or entered, even as it installs in the world the dream of occupying that outside. So if death is always punctual, dying always has the form of a sentence—and if dying is a ceaseless murmur, that murmur is nonetheless bent over and over again to the particular periods, gaps, and caesuras that make that murmur something other than mere noise. It is in this mutual scansion that death is of the world and does not hold itself beyond representation except by also being held within it. And so it participates in more general vicissitudes of representation. That it does so is part and parcel of its singularity. One cannot ask that death be withheld from representation or that there be no politics of dying, but only that that politics not fail to mark what it is of—a marking that may make of it something more or less or other than a politics and that will, in the end, determine what it is to speak of an AIDS community as it determines what it might mean to speak of any community. Here too it matters to insert a comma, to register the gap—the nothing—that gives the two words and the two things their solidarity.

Blanchot cites Bataille: No one has the right not to belong to my absence of community. No higher logic intervenes to redeem this string of negatives, to gather up what it disperses into a positive community that might then affirm itself on the ground of a common humanity, and so Bataille's readers are left to find their way in relation to an absence from which they can neither be excluded nor exclude themselves. And yet Bataille, and Blanchot citing him, clearly mean this to count as a way toward the acknowledgment of how we are with one another. If they are successful in this, it will be because, right failing, we find ourselves faced with the prospect of a naked and unsecured obligation to that absence, an obligation that picks us out, one by one, in our singularity.

Yingling, Tom

I would like to believe that in saying these things I am saying something not wholly foreign to the shape of Tom's intrigue with Wittgenstein and national bodies and the abrupt emergence of Bataille in his consideration of filmic responses to AIDS. But, in the end, nothing of that kind can authorize my words: I can claim no shared theoretical posture with him, as I can also claim no common sexuality, no shared suffering, no mutual activism, and no deep friendship. We got along well and promised one another more time and never found it—so in the end we shared a stretch of time and space and friends and little more. I have, I dare say, no right to speak of him, and I imagine the absence of that right to be legible in the turns of grammatical person— first and third, singular and plural—that variously mark, elide, or efface a voice that can claim securely neither anonymity nor the urgency of subjectivity, personal or sheerly human, for itself. Almost nothing, then—a voice attempting to read, too late and under the obscurest of obligations, the rhythm of a friendship unaccomplished.

Names, too, are in their way clichés. On the occasion of death, but also in the order of our institutional lives, we often break and reform them, laying straight the lines of filiation and reshaping their apparent empty repetition as species and genus: Yingling, Thomas, finds its place on the roll of the dead and in our bibliographies. Criticism, it seems to me, works otherwise. It hears in the name something at once solid and fissured with inscription, twisting repetition and heterogeneity, repeating the self in otherness; a form, paradigm, or ruined stereotype of community. What it wants, its way of having and letting go, is to hear the text repeated in its separation from itself: Tom, then—Tom, Yingling

Bibliography

Abraham, Julie. "I Know What Boys Like: Tales from the Dyke Side." *Village Voice Literary Supplement* (June 1992): 20–23.

Adorno, Theodor. *Notes to Literature.* 1958. Ed. Rolf Tiedemann. Trans. Shierry Weber Nicholsen. Vol I. New York: Columbia UP, 1991.

——. *Prisms.* 1967. Trans. Samuel and Shierry Weber. Cambridge: MIT Press, 1986.

"Age of AIDS: A Death in the Family." *Village Voice* 23 Mar. 1993: 13.

"AIDS: Grin and Bear It, a New Humor Magazine." *Newsweek* 15 Apr. 1991: 58.

Alexander, Benita, and Lorenzo Benet. "Believe in Magic." *People Weekly* 25 Nov. 1991: 59.

Alonso, Ana Maria, and Maria Teresa Koreck. "Silences: 'Hispanics,' AIDS, and Sexual Practices." *differences* 1.1 (Winter 1989): 101–24.

Althusser, Louis. "Ideology and Ideological State Apparatuses (Notes Towards an Investigation)." *Lenin and Philosophy and Other Essays.* Trans. Ben Brewster. New York: Monthly Review, 1971. 121–73.

Arac, Jonathan. "F. O. Matthiessen: Authorizing an American Renaissance." *The American Renaissance Reconsidered.* Ed. Walter B. Michaels and Donald E. Pease. Baltimore: Johns Hopkins UP, 1985. 90–112.

Arendt, Hannah. *The Origins of Totalitarianism.* New York: Harcourt Brace Jovanovich, 1951.

Asante, Molefi Kete. *The Afrocentric Idea.* Philadelphia: Temple UP, 1987.

Ashbery, John. *Selected Poems.* New York: Viking, 1985.

"Back to the Bad Old Days." *Time* 20 May 1991: 28.

Bad Object-Choices, ed. *How Do I Look? Queer Film and Video.* Seattle: Bay, 1991.

Bakhtin, M. M. "Discourse in the Novel." *The Dialogic Imagination: Four Essays.* Ed. Michael Holquist. Trans. Caryl Emerson and Michael Holquist. Austin: U of Texas P, 1981. 259–422.

Barthes, Roland. *Camera Lucida.* 1980. Trans. Richard Howard. New York: Farrar, Straus, and Giroux, 1981.

——. *Mythologies.* 1957. Trans. Annette Lavers. New York: Noonday, 1992.

Baudrillard, Jean. *In the Shadow of the Silent Majorities.* 1978. Trans. Paul Foss, Paul Patton, and John Johnston. New York: Semiotext(e), 1983.

Beaches. Dir. Garry Marshall. Touchstone Pictures, 1988.

Benfey, Christopher. "Telling It Slant." *New Republic* 18 Mar. 1991: 40.

Benjamin, Walter. *Illuminations.* Ed. Hannah Arendt. Trans. Harry Zohn. New York: Schocken Books, 1969.

Bennett, Tony. *Formalism and Marxism.* London: Methuen, 1979.

Bercovitch, Sacvan. *The American Jeremiad.* Madison: U of Wisconsin P, 1978.

Bercovitch, Sacvan, and Myra Jehlen, eds. *Ideology and Classic American Literature.* New York: Cambridge UP, 1986.

Berlant, Lauren. "National Brands/National Body: *Imitation of Life.*" *Comparative American Identities: Race, Sex, and Nationality in the Modern Text.* Ed. Hortense Spillers. New York: Routledge, 1991. 110–40.

Bersani, Leo. *Homos.* Cambridge, MA, and London: Harvard UP, 1995.

——. "Is the Rectum a Grave?" *October* 43 (Winter 1987): 197–222.

Bhabha, Homi. "The Other Question: The Stereotype and Colonial Discourse." *Screen* 24 (Nov.–Dec. 1983): 18–36.

Bourdieu, Pierre. *In Other Words: Essays Toward a Reflexive Sociology.* Trans. Matthew Adamson. Stanford: Stanford UP, 1990.

"Bumbling Toward the Nobel." *Time* 20 May 1991: 50.

Burgin, Victor. "Photographic Practice and Art Theory." *Thinking Photography.* Ed. Victor Burgin. London: Macmillan, 1982. 39–83.

Butler, Judith. "The Force of Fantasy: Feminism, Mapplethorpe, and Discursive Excess." *differences* 2.2 (1990): 105–25.

——. *Gender Trouble: Feminism and the Subversion of Identity.* New York: Routledge, 1990.

——. "Gender Trouble, Feminist Theory, and Psychoanalytic Discourse." *Feminism/Postmodernism.* Ed. Linda Nicholson. New York: Routledge, 1990: 324–40.

——. "Letter to the Editor." *NYQ* 12 Apr. 1992.

Butters, Ronald R. "Foreword." *Displacing Homophobia. South Atlantic Quarterly* (special issue) 88.1 (Winter 1989): 1–5.

Califa, Pat. "Feminism and Sadomasochism." *Heresies* 3.4 (1981): 30–34.

——. "Unraveling the Sexual Fringe: A Secret Side of Lesbian Sexuality." *The Advocate* 27 Dec. 1979: 19–23.

Case, Sue-Ellen. "The Student and the Strap: Authority and Seduction in the Class/Room." *Professions of Desire.* Ed. George Haggerty and Bonnie Zimmerman. New York: MLA Publications, 1995. 38–46.

Clifford, James. *The Predicament of Culture: Twentieth-Century Ethnography, Literature, and Art.* Cambridge: Harvard UP, 1988.

Cohen, Ed. "Are We (Not) What We Are Becoming? 'Gay' 'Identity,' 'Gay Studies,' and the Disciplining of Knowledge." *Engendering Men: The Question of Male Feminist Criticism.* Ed. Joseph Boone and Michael Cadden. New York: Routledge, 1990. 161–75.

Creech, James. *Closet Writing/Gay Reading: The Case of Melville's Pierre.* Chicago: U of Chicago P, 1993.

Crimp, Douglas, ed. *AIDS: Cultural Analysis/Cultural Activism.* Cambridge: MIT P, 1988.

——. "Art Acts Up." *Out/Look* 9 (Summer 1990): 22–30.

——. "Right On, Girlfriend!" *Social Text* 33 (1992): 2–19.

Crimp, Douglas, with Adam Rolston. *AIDS Demo Graphics.* Seattle: Bay, 1990.

de Lauretis, Teresa. *The Practice of Love: Lesbian Sexuality and Perverse Desire.* Bloomington: Indiana UP, 1994.

"Delays That Can Cause Death." *Time* 4 Feb. 1991: 69.

de Man, Paul. "Conclusions: Walter Benjamin's 'Task of the Translator.' " *The Resistance to Theory.* Minneapolis: U of Minnesota P, 1986. 73–105.

D'Emilio, John. *Making Trouble: Essays on Gay History, Politics, and the University.* New York: Routledge, 1992.

Derrida, Jacques. *Of Grammatology.* 1967. Trans. Gayatri Chakravorty Spivak. Baltimore: Johns Hopkins UP, 1976.

"Desert Victory." *Newsweek* 18 Mar. 1991: 22.

Dickinson, Emily. "There's a certain Slant of light." *The Complete Poems of Emily Dickinson.* Ed. Thomas H. Johnson. Boston and Toronto: Little, Brown, 1960. 118.

Displacing Homophobia. Ed. Ronald R. Butters, John M. Clum, and Michael Moon. *South Atlantic Quarterly* (special issue) 88.1 (Winter 1989).

Dollimore, Jonathan. "Different Desires: Subjectivity and Transgression in Wilde and Gide." *Genders* 2 (Summer 1990): 24–41.

Duberman, Martin. Interview by M. L. Cooper. *Lambda Book Report* 3.8 (1993): 10–11.

Duberman, Martin, Martha Vicinus, and George Chauncey, Jr., eds. *Hidden from History: Reclaiming the Gay and Lesbian Past.* New York: NAL Books, 1989.

Dulles, John Foster. *War or Peace.* New York: Macmillan, 1950.

Dunne, Dominick. "Interview with Mapplethorpe." *Vanity Fair* Feb. 1989: 126+.

Dworkin, Andrea. *Pornography: Men Possessing Women.* New York: Putnam's, 1979.

An Early Frost. Dir. John Erman. 1985.

Easton, Richard. "Canonical Criminalizations: Homosexuality, Art History, Surrealism, and Abjection." *differences* 4.3 (Fall 1992): 133–75.

Edelman, Lee. "At Risk in the Sublime: The Politics of Gender and Theory." *Gender and Theory: Dialogues on Feminist Criticism.* Ed. Linda Kauffman. London: Basil Blackwell, 1989. 213–24.

——. *Homographesis: Essays in Gay Literary and Cultural Theory.* New York and London: Routledge, 1994.

——. "The Plague of Discourse: Politics, Literary Theory, and AIDS." *South Atlantic Quarterly* 88.1 (Winter 1989): 301–17.

Eliot, T. S. *The Waste Land, and Other Poems.* New York: Harcourt Brace, 1958. 1958.

Ellis, John. "On Pornography." *Screen* 21.1 (Spring 1980): 81–108.

Epps, Brad. "Sense and Sensibility: Eros, Pedagogy, and (In)discretion in Ana Maria Moix, Esther Tusquets, and Carme Riera." Paper presented at "Gender, Sexuality, and the State: A Latino/Hispanic Context Conference." U of California-Berkeley, 1993.

Escoffier, Jeffrey. "Inside the Ivory Closet: The Challenges Facing Lesbian and Gay Studies." *Out/Look* (Fall 1990): 40–48.

Fisher, Andrea. *Let Us Now Praise Famous Women.* London: Pandora, 1987.

"The Fog of War." *Time* 4 Feb. 1991: 16.

Foucault, Michel. *The History of Sexuality: An Introduction.* 1978. Trans. Robert Hurley. New York: Vintage Books, 1990.

Frank, Robert. *The Americans.* New York: SCALO Publishers, 1959.

Fukuyama, Francis. "The End of History?" *The National Interest* 16 (Summer 1989): 3–18.

Fuss, Diana. *Essentially Speaking: Feminism, Nature and Difference.* New York: Routledge, 1989.

——, ed. *Inside/Out: Lesbian Theories, Gay Theories.* New York: Routledge, 1991.

"The Future of Gay America." *Newsweek* 12 Mar. 1990: 20–27.

Gilbert, Sandra, and Susan Gubar. "The Man on the Dump vs the United Dames of America; or What Does Mr. Lentricchia Want?" *Critical Inquiry* 14 (Winter 1988): 386–406.

——, eds. *The Norton Anthology of Literature by Women.* New York: W. W. Norton, 1985.

Gilman, Sander. "Black Bodies, White Bodies: Toward an Iconography of Female Sexuality in Late Nineteenth Century Art, Medicine, and Literature." *"Race," Writing and Difference.* Ed. Henry Louis Gates, Jr. Chicago: U of Chicago P, 1985. 223–61.

Greenberg, David E. *The Construction of Homosexuality.* Chicago: U of Chicago P, 1988.

Greenblatt, Stephen. *Shakespearean Negotiations: The Circulation of Social Energy in Renaissance England.* Berkeley: U of California P, 1988.

"Grief Counseling for Colleagues of AIDS Victims." *Newsweek* 7 Jan. 1991: 61.

Griffin, Susan. *Pornography and Silence: Culture's Revenge against Nature.* New York: Harper, 1982.

Grosz, Elizabeth. "Bodies and Pleasures in Queer Theory." *Who Can Speak? Authority and Critical Identity.* Ed. Judith Roof and Robyn Wiegman. Urbana: U of Illinois P, 1995. 221–30.

Grover, Jan Zita. "AIDS: Key-words." *October* 43 (Winter 1987): 17–30.

Gunn, Thom. *Collected Poems.* New York: Noonday, 1994.

Habermas, Jürgen. "Modernity—An Incomplete Project." *The Anti-Aesthetic: Essays on Postmodern Culture.* Ed. Hal Foster. Seattle: Bay, 1983. 3–15.

Haggerty, George, and Bonnie Zimmerman, eds. *Professions of Desire: Gay and Lesbian Studies in Literature.* New York: MLA Publications, 1995.

Haraway, Donna. "The Biopolitics of Postmodern Bodies: Determination of Self in Immune System Discourse." *differences* 1.1 (Winter 1989): 3–43.

Harper, Philip Brian. "Eloquence and Epitaph: Black Nationalism and the Homophobic Impulse in Responses to the Death of Max Robinson." *Writing AIDS: Gay Literature, Language, and Analysis.* Ed. Timothy F. Murphy and Suzanne Poirier. New York: Columbia UP, 1993. 117–39.

Hay, Louise. *The AIDS Book: Creating a Positive Approach.* Santa Monica, CA: Hay House, 1988.

Hemphill, Essex, ed. *Brother to Brother: New Writing by Black Gay Men.* New York: Alyson Publications, 1991.

Hertz, Neil. "The Notion of Blockage in the Literature of the Sublime." *The End of the Line: Essays on Psychoanalysis and the Sublime.* New York: Columbia UP, 1985. 40–60.

Hurston, Zora Neale. *Their Eyes Were Watching God.* 1937. Urbana: U of Illinois P, 1978.

Irigaray, Luce. *This Sex Which Is Not One.* 1977. Trans. Catherine Porter with Carolyn Burke. Ithaca: Cornell UP, 1985.

Ischar, Doug. "Household Misappropriations." Visual Studies Workshop Exhibit, Rochester, New York, Spring 1989.

Jameson, Fredric. "Pleasure: A Political Issue." *The Ideologies of Theory: Essays 1971–1986. Volume 2: The Syntax of History.* Minneapolis: U of Minnesota P, 1988. 61–74.

Jones, Gayl. *Corregidora.* 1975. Boston: Beacon, 1986.

Joselit, David. "Robert Mapplethorpe's Poses." *Robert Mapplethorpe: The Perfect Moment.* Ed. Janet Kardon. Philadelphia: Institute of Contemporary Art, 1991. 19–21.

Julien, Isaac, and Kobena Mercer. "True Confessions: A Discourse on Images of Black Male Sexuality." *Ten.8* 22 (1986): 4–8.

Kaplan, Cora. "Pandora's Box: Subjectivity, Class and Sexuality in Socialist Feminist Criticism." *Making A Difference: Feminist Literary Criticism.* Ed. Gayle Greene and Coppelia Kahn. London: Methuen, 1985. 146–76.

Kaplan, E. Ann. "Pornography and/as Representation." *enclitic 17/18* 9.1–2 (1987): 8–19.

Kardon, Janet. "The Perfect Moment." *Robert Mapplethorpe: The Perfect Moment.* Ed. Janet Kardon. Philadelphia: Institute of Contemporary Art, 1991. 9–13.

———. "Robert Mapplethorpe Interview." *Robert Mapplethorpe: The Perfect Moment.* Ed. Janet Kardon. Philadelphia: Institute of Contemporary Art, 1991. 23–29.

Kibbey, Ann. *The Interpretation of Material Shapes in Puritanism: A Study of Rhetoric, Prejudice, and Violence.* Cambridge and New York: Cambridge UP, 1986.

Kimball, Roger. "'Heterosexuality' and Other Literary Matters." *Wall Street Journal* 31 Dec. 1992: A6.

Kinsella, James. *Covering the Plague: AIDS and the American Media.* New Brunswick: Rutgers UP, 1989.

Kozol, Wendy. "Madonnas of the Fields: Photography, Gender, and 1930s Farm Relief." *Genders* 2 (Summer 1988): 1–23.

Kushner, Tony. *Angels in America, Part 1: Millennium Approaches.* New York: Theatre Communications Group, 1993.

Lacan, Jacques. *The Four Fundamental Concepts of Psycho-Analysis.* 1973. Ed. Jacques-Alain Miller. Trans. Alan Sheridan. New York: W. W. Norton, 1981.

Laclau, Ernesto, and Chantel Mouffe. *Hegemony and Socialist Strategy: Towards a Radical Democratic Politics.* London: Verso, 1985.

Larson, Kay. "Robert Mapplethorpe." *Robert Mapplethorpe: The Perfect Moment.* Ed. Janet Kardon. Philadelphia: Institute of Contemporary Art, 1991. 15–17.

Lentricchia, Frank. "Patriarchy Against Itself—The Young Manhood of Wallace Stevens." *Critical Inquiry* 13.4 (Summer 1987): 742–86.

Leo, John. "The Familialism of 'Man' in American Television Melodrama." *South Atlantic Quarterly* 88.1 (Winter 1989): 31–52.

Lesbian and Gay Studies Newsletter. Winter 1989.

Levinson, Marjorie. "The New Historicism: Back to the Future." *Rethinking Historicism: Cultural Reading in Romantic History.* Ed. Marjorie Levinson, Marilyn Butler, Jerome McGann, and Paul Hamilton. Oxford and New York: Basil Blackwell, 1989. 18–63.

——. *Wordsworth's Great Period Poems: Four Essays.* Cambridge and New York: Cambridge UP, 1986.

Litvak, Joseph. "Teaching and Melancholia." Paper presented at the Modern Language Association Conference. New York, 1993.

Longtime Companion. Dir. Norman Rene. Samuel Goldwyn, 1990.

Looking for Langston. Dir. Isaac Julien. Frameline, 1989.

Lowell, Robert. *Life Studies and For the Union Dead.* New York: Farrar, Straus, and Giroux, 1964.

Lyotard, Jean-François. "Discussions, or Phrasing 'after Auschwitz.'" Trans. Georges Van Den Abbeele. Working Paper No. 2, Fall 1986. Milwaukee: Center for Twentieth Century Studies, 1986. 16–27.

——. *The Post-Modern Condition: A Report on Knowledge.* 1979. Trans. Geoff Bennington and Brian Massumi. Minneapolis: U of Minnesota P, 1984.

MacLeish, Archibald. *Conquistador.* New York: Houghton Mifflin, 1932.

Mapplethorpe, Robert. *Black Book.* New York: St. Martin's, 1986.

Martin, Wendy. *An American Triptych: Anne Bradstreet, Emily Dickinson, Adrienne Rich.* Chapel Hill: U of North Carolina P, 1984.

Mathy, Jean-Phillipe. "Out of History: French Readings of Postmodern America." *American Literary History* 2.2 (Summer 1990): 267–98.

Matthiessen, Francis Otto. *American Renaissance: Art and Expression in the Age of Emerson and Whitman.* London: Oxford UP, 1941.

——. *Rat and the Devil: Journal Letters of F. O. Matthiessen and Russell Cheney.* Ed. Louis Hyde. Hamden, CT: Archon, 1978.

Mercer, Kobena. "Imaging the Black Men's Sex." *Photography—Politics, Two.* Ed. Patricia Holland, Jo Spence, and Simon Watney. London: Camedia, 1987. n. pag.

Michaels, Walter Benn, and Donald E. Pease, eds. *The American Renaissance Reconsidered.* Baltimore: Johns Hopkins UP, 1985.

Miller, D. A. "*Cage aux Folles:* Sensation and Gender in Wilkie Collins's *The Woman in White.*" *The Making of the Modern Body: Sexuality and Society in the Nineteenth Century.* Ed. Catherine Gallagher and Thomas Laquer. Berkeley: U of California P, 1987. 107–36.

——. *The Novel and the Police.* Berkeley: U of California P, 1988.

Millett, Kate. *Sexual Politics.* New York: Ballantine Books, 1969.

Mohr, Richard. *Gay Ideas: Outing and Other Controversies.* Boston: Beacon, 1992.

Monette, Paul. *Becoming a Man: Half a Life Story.* New York: Harcourt Brace Jovanovich, 1992.

——. *Borrowed Time: An AIDS Memoir.* New York: Harcourt Brace Jovanovich, 1988.

Moon, Michael, and Eve Kosofsky Sedgwick. "Divinity: A Dossier: A Performance Piece: A Little-Understood Emotion." *Discourse* 13.1 (Fall–Winter 1990–91): 12–39.

Morrison, Toni. *Beloved.* New York: Signet, 1987.

——. *Sula.* New York: Bantam, 1973.

Nussbaum, Martha. "A Classical Case for Gay Studies." *New Republic* 13 and 20 July 1992: 26–35.

"On the Fence." *Time* 14 Jan. 1991: 12.

Other Countries: Black Gay Men Writing Collective. *Acquired Visions: Seeing Ourselves Through AIDS.* Performance. The Underground. Syracuse, NY. 9 Feb. 1990.

Outweek: The Lesbian and Gay News Magazine. 27 Feb. 1991.

Paris Is Burning. Dir. Jennie Livingston. Academy Entertainment, 1991.

Parting Glances. Dir. Bill Sherwood. Rondo Pictures, 1985.

Patrick, Robert. "Letter." *Out/Look* 1.4 (Winter 1989): 6.

Patton, Cindy. *Inventing AIDS.* New York: Routledge, 1990.

Perloff, Marjorie. "Canon and Loaded Gun: Feminist Poetics and the Avant-Garde." *Stanford Literature Review* 4.1 (Spring 1987): 23–46.

Phillips, Sandra S. "A Body of Work (on Johns Coplans)." Exhibit at the Art Institute of Chicago, April 1989.

Pink Flamingoes. Dir. John Waters. Dreamland Productions, 1972.

Plath, Sylvia. *Ariel.* New York: Harper and Row, 1961.

——. *The Colossus and Other Poems.* New York: Vintage Books, 1957.

Poison. Dir. Todd Haynes. Bronze Eye Productions, 1991.

Pokorny, Sydney. "The Root of My Obsession with Sandra and Madonna Is Unbridled Lust." *Gay Community News* 17.4 (30 July–5 Aug. 1989): 10.

Rampersad, Arnold. *The Life of Langston Hughes.* 2 vols. New York: Oxford UP, 1986–88.

Renza, Louis. *"A White Heron" and the Question of Minor Literature.* Madison: U of Wisconsin P, 1984.

Rich, Adrienne. "Rape." *Diving into the Wreck: Poems 1971–1972.* New York: W. W. Norton, 1973. 44–45.

Riggs, Marlon. "Unleash the Queen." *Black Popular Culture.* Ed. Gina Dent. Seattle: Bay, 1993. 99–105.

Román, David. "Teaching Differences: Theory and Practice in a Lesbian and Gay Studies Seminar." *Professions of Desire.* Ed. George Haggerty and Bonnie Zimmerman. New York: MLA Publications, 1995. 113–23.

Roof, Judith. *A Lure of Knowledge: Lesbian Sexuality and Theory.* New York: Columbia UP, 1991.

"Saddam's Endgame." *Newsweek* 7 Jan. 1991: 14–26.

"Saddam's Slaughter." *Newsweek* 15 Apr. 1991: 22.

Sedgwick, Eve Kosofsky. "Across Gender, Across Sexuality: Willa Cather and Others." *South Atlantic Quarterly* 88.1 (Winter 1989): 53–72.

——. *Between Men: English Literature and Male Homosocial Desire.* New York: Columbia UP, 1985.

——. *Epistemology of the Closet.* Berkeley: U of California P, 1990.

——. "White Glasses." *Yale Journal of Criticism* 5 (1992): 193–208.

Sekula, Allan. "On the Invention of Photographic Meaning." *Thinking Photography.* Ed. Victor Burgin. London: Macmillan, 1982. 84–109.

Shilts, Randy. *And the Band Played On: Politics, People, and the AIDS Epidemic.* New York: St. Martin's, 1987.

The Silence of the Lambs. Dir. Jonathan Demme. Orion Pictures, 1991.

Smith, Barbara. "Toward a Black Feminist Criticism." *The New Feminist Criticism.* Ed. Elaine Showalter. New York: Pantheon, 1985. 168–85.

Sontag, Susan. *AIDS and Its Metaphors.* New York: Farrar, Straus, and Giroux, 1988.

Stein, Gertrude. *How Writing Is Written.* Ed. Robert Bartlett Haas. Los Angeles: Black Sparrow, 1974.

Stevens, Wallace. "Notes Toward a Supreme Fiction." *The Collected Poems.* New York: Random House, 1954. 380–408.

Sullivan, Andrew. "Gay Life, Gay Death." *New Republic* 17 Dec. 1990: 19–25.

Tagg, John. "The Currency of the Photography." *Thinking Photography.* Ed. Victor Burgin. London: Macmillan, 1982. 110–41.

Taylor, John. "Are You Politically Correct?" *New York* 21 Jan. 1991: 32–40.

"A Tempest in the Test Tube." *Newsweek* 18 Mar. 1991: 48.

Theweleit, Klaus. *Male Fantasies.* 1977. Trans. Stephen Conway. 2 vols. Minneapolis: U of Minnesota P, 1987–89.

Tongues Untied. Dir. Marlon Riggs. Frameline, 1989.

Turner, Victor. *The Ritual Process: Structure and Anti-Structure.* New York: Aldine, 1969.

Untermeyer, Louis, ed. *The Poetry and Prose of Walt Whitman.* New York: Simon and Schuster, 1949.

Warner, Michael. "From Queer to Eternity: An Army of Theorists Cannot Fail." *Village Voice Supplement* June 1992: 18–19.

——. "Walden's Erotic Economy." *Comparative American Identities: Race, Sex, and Nationality in the Modern Text.* Ed. Hortense Spillers. New York: Routledge, 1991. 157–74.

Watney, Simon. "Lesbian and Gay Studies in the Age of AIDS." *NYQ* 22 Mar. 1992: 42.

——. "Missionary Positions: AIDS, 'Africa,' and Race." *differences* 1.1 (Winter 1989): 83–101.

——. *Policing Desire: Pornography, AIDS, and the Media.* Minneapolis: U of Minnesota P, 1987.

Weber, Bruce. *O Rio de Janeiro.* New York: Knopf, 1986.

Weeks, Jeffrey. *Sexuality and Its Discontents: Meanings, Myths, and Modern Sexualities.* London: Routledge and Kegan Paul, 1985.

"When the Doctor Gets Infected." *Time* 14 Jan. 1991: 57.

Wiegman, Robyn. "Negotiating the Masculine." Diss. U of Washington, 1988.

Will, George. "Literary Politics." *Newsweek* 22 Apr. 1991: 72.

Wittgenstein, Ludwig. *Culture and Value*. 1931. Trans. Peter Winch. Chicago: U of Chicago P, 1980.

Wolf, Larry. "Letter." *Out/Look* 1.4 (Winter 1989): 5.

Wyschogrod, Edith. *Spirit in Ashes: Hegel, Heidegger, and Man-Made Mass Death*. New Haven: Yale UP, 1985.

Yarbro-Bejarano, Yvonne. "Expanding the Categories of Race and Sexuality in Lesbian and Gay Studies." *Professions of Desire*. Ed. George Haggerty and Bonnie Zimmerman. New York: MLA Publications, 1995. 125–35.

Yingling, Thomas E. *Hart Crane and the Homosexual Text: New Thresholds, New Anatomies*. Chicago: U of Chicago P, 1990.

Yúdice, George. "Marginality and the Ethics of Survival." *Universal Abandon? The Politics of Postmodernism*. Ed. Andrew Ross. Minneapolis: U of Minnesota P, 1988. 214–36.

Index

Contributors

Michael Awkward is Professor of English and Afro-American and African Studies at the University of Michigan. His most recent book is *Negotiating Difference,* published by University of Chicago Press.

Robert L. Caserio directs graduate studies in English at Temple University. His most recent essays are "Queer Passion, Queer Citizenship" in *Modern Fiction Studies* (Spring 1997) and "Casement, Joyce and Pound" in *Queer Joyce* (University of Michigan Press). He has just completed *The English Novel 1900–1950* (forthcoming from Twayne Macmillan) and is at work on *Citizen Queer: Anglo-American Fiction and Democratic Dogmas in the Twentieth Century.*

Stephen Melville, a former member of the English department faculty at Syracuse University, is currently Associate Professor of Art History at Ohio State University. He is the author of *Philosophy Beside Itself* (Minnesota) and *Seams: Art as a Philosophical Context* (Gordon & Breach), and co-editor of *Vision and Textuality* with Bill Readings (Macmillan).

David Román is Assistant Professor of English at the University of Southern California. His book, *Acts of Intervention: Gay Men, U.S. Theatre, AIDS* is forthcoming from Indiana University Press. He serves on the editorial board of *GLQ: A Journal of Gay and Lesbian Studies.*

Robyn Wiegman, a former member of the English department at Syracuse University, now directs the Women's Studies Program at the University of California-Irvine. She has published *American Anatomies: Theorizing Race and Gender* (Duke, 1995) and coedited two volumes, *Who Can Speak? Authority and Critical Identity* and *Feminism Beside Itself.*

Thomas E. Yingling was Associate Professor of English and Director of Graduate Studies at Syracuse University at the time of his death in 1992. Author of *Hart Crane and the Homosexual Text* (University of Chicago 1990), he received his Ph.D. from the University of Pennsylvania.

Acknowledgment of Copyrights

"Wittgenstein's Tumor: AIDS and the National Body," *Textual Practice* 8.1 (Spring 1994): 97–113. Used with the permission of Routledge Press.

"AIDS in America: Postmodern Governance, Identity, and Experience," *Inside/Out: Lesbian Theories, Gay Theories,* ed. Diana Fuss (New York: Routledge, 1991): 291–310. Used with the permission of Routledge Press.

"How the Eye is Caste: Robert Mapplethorpe and the Limits of Controversy," *Discourse* 12.2 (Spring–Summer 1990): 3–28.

"Sexual Preference/Cultural Reference: The Predicament of Gay Culture Studies," excerpted from *American Literary History* 3.1 (Spring 1991): 184–96. Used with the permission of Oxford University Press.

"Fetishism, Identity, Politics," originally appeared in *Who Can Speak? Identity and Critical Authority,* ed. Judith Roof and Robyn Wiegman (Urbana: University of Illinois Press, 1995): 155–64. Copyright 1995 by the Board of Trustees of the University of Illinois. Used with the permission of the University of Illinois Press.

"Speaking with the Dead," originally appeared in *Who Can Speak? Identity and Critical Authority,* ed. Judith Roof and Robyn Wiegman (Urbana: University of Illinois Press, 1995): 165–79. Copyright 1995 by the Board of Trustees of the University of Illinois. Used with the permission of the University of Illinois Press.

Library of Congress Cataloging-in-Publication Data
Yingling, Thomas E.
AIDS and the national body /
edited with an introduction by Robyn Wiegman.
p.   cm. — (Series Q)
Includes bibliographical references and index.
ISBN 0-8223-1977-2 (alk. paper). — ISBN 0-8223-1973-X (pbk. : alk. paper)
1. AIDS (Disease)—Social aspects—United States.
I. Wiegman, Robyn.   II. Series.
RA644.A25Y56   1997   362.1'969792'00973—
dc21   96-40282 CIP